Therapists' Guide to Overcoming Grief and Loss After Brain Injury

Therapists' Guide to Overcoming Grief and Loss After Brain Injury

Janet P. Niemeier • Robert L. Karol

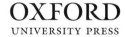
UNIVERSITY PRESS

2011

OXFORD
UNIVERSITY PRESS

Oxford University Press, Inc., publishes works that further
Oxford University's objective of excellence
in research, scholarship, and education.

Oxford   New York
Auckland   Cape Town   Dar es Salaam   Hong Kong   Karachi
Kuala Lumpur   Madrid   Melbourne   Mexico City   Nairobi
New Delhi   Shanghai   Taipei   Toronto

With offices in
Argentina   Austria   Brazil   Chile   Czech Republic   France   Greece
Guatemala   Hungary   Italy   Japan   Poland   Portugal   Singapore
South Korea   Switzerland   Thailand   Turkey   Ukraine   Vietnam

Copyright © 2011 by Oxford University Press, Inc.

Published by Oxford University Press, Inc.
198 Madison Avenue, New York, New York 10016

www.oup.com

Oxford is a registered trademark of Oxford University Press

All rights reserved. No part of this publication may be reproduced,
stored in a retrieval system, or transmitted, in any form or by any means,
electronic, mechanical, photocopying, recording, or otherwise,
without the prior permission of Oxford University Press.

Library of Congress Cataloging-in-Publication Data

Niemeier, Janet P., 1947–
    Therapist's guide to overcoming grief & loss after brain injury / Janet P. Niemeier, Robert L. Karol.
       p. ; cm.
    Other title: Therapist's guide to overcoming grief and loss after brain injury
    Companion volume to: Overcoming grief and loss after brain injury / Janet P. Niemeier, Robert L. Karol. 2011.
    Includes bibliographical references and index.
    ISBN 978-0-19-538896-1   1. Brain damage—Patients—Rehabilitation.   2. Brain damage—Psychological aspects.
3. Grief.   4. Loss (Psychology)   I. Karol, Robert L.   II. Niemeier, Janet P., 1947–. Overcoming grief and loss
after brain injury.   III. Title. IV. Title: Therapist's guide to overcoming grief and loss after brain injury.
    [DNLM: 1. Brain Injuries—rehabilitation—Handbooks.   2. Brain Injuries—psychology—Handbooks.
3. Psychotherapy—methods—Handbooks.   4. Stress, Psychological—rehabilitation—Handbooks.   WL 39 N672t 2011]
    RC387.5.N543 2011
    617.4'81044—dc22
                                                                                                                                2010015045

ISBN-13: 9780195388961

9 8 7 6 5 4 3 2 1
Printed in the United States of America
on acid-free paper

To Betty and Bob for giving me an early life that allowed me to love diversity and appreciate differences, and to Dave, Carrie, Clay, and Carolyn, my wonderful family, who love and support me always and put up with my preoccupations.

—JPN

To Rhona, for whom I will always grieve, and to Gwen, who helps me survive everything: We are a team forever and ever.

—RLK

Preface

When people present to professionals grieving loss, providers are often uncertain as to how to proceed. There are known protocols and treatment pathways for depression, anxiety, etc., both through psychotherapy and medication. Not so with grief, particularly after brain injury.

People are generally unprepared for hospital rehabilitation. Moreover, while medical advances are keeping more people alive following brain injury, health care coverage and lengths of hospital stays are shrinking so that optimal rehabilitation is not always available for persons with brain injury and there is not enough time to grieve. People with brain injury are getting discharged to the community very quickly. Now lengths of stay are measured in days and weeks and no longer months. There is insufficient time to help people learn to respond to having a brain injury. Many people are not emotionally ready and are still experiencing significant grief at hospital discharge. Also, they often arrive back home with significant levels of impairment in cognition and functional skills. Furthermore, outpatient services are frequently fragmented or beyond people's means to access.

Hence, there are two problems: inadequate time in rehabilitation and disjointed follow-up care. Both make grieving much harder. This in turn leaves people with brain injury at a loss to find their emotional way. The companion book to this one, written for people with brain injuries, *Overcoming Grief and Loss After Brain Injury,* was written to help people respond to brain injury. *Therapist's Guide to Overcoming Grief and Loss After Brain Injury* was written to help you guide the people who seek your advice.

The intent is to help you convey hope and coping strategies. We believe that persons with brain injury can respond to brain injury successfully. Note that we said "respond," not adjust, since we believe that this is an ongoing process, whereas "adjust" implies finality. Learning to respond is part of life and we are ardent believers in the capacity of persons with brain injury to respond.

Janet P. Niemeier
Robert L. Karol

Acknowledgments

I have learned from many hundreds of my clients with brain injury how little there is out there in terms of practical resources to help people with brain injury and their families adjust to this complicated and challenging injury. I hope the book will provide a strong foundation of information and coping skills as well as a guide for not only clients with brain injury but their therapists who want to help them. Thanks to all of you for giving me the gift of sharing your experiences and selves for a little of your journey.

I am grateful and want to thank all of my mentors at Virginia Commonwealth University Health System Brain Injury Unit, Outpatient Neuropsychology and Rehabilitation Psychology Services, the Rehabilitation and Research Center on North Hospital First Floor at VCUHS, and in Egyptian. I have learned skills, patience, sensitivity, and empathy from you all. Without your modeling and support I would not have been able to reach this point.

My deep admiration goes to many wonderful colleagues tackling the difficult issues on the community front line where fragmented services for persons with brain injury lead you toward creativity, amazing advocacy, and self-sacrifice that I have noted and tried to emulate.

To the staff of Oxford, I am grateful for your confidence in us and support of this project which will hopefully help many persons and their families who did not ask for but are trying their best to live with this injury and its aftermath.

To my brother, Tim, and his family, Mary, Chris, Thomas, Chrystal, and the new generation represented by Lucas. I am proud of you all and grateful for your being out there in the world for me to love and as my family of supporters.

Most of all, thanks to my Richmond, Virginia and Ypsilanti, Michigan family—Dave, Carrie, Clay, Carolyn, and Patrick—who love and are with me no matter what. I could not do anything without you. Thanks to Raleigh for pointing out that it is important to take a break and play catch sometimes.

—JPN

Foremost in my thoughts as I wrote this book were the persons with brain injury and their families with whom I have worked over all of my years of practice. I have learned so much from them that I have shared with other people grieving their own losses. I have always explained to newly injured people that the role of the therapist is to be a conduit of knowledge from the past successes and setbacks of previous clients to newly injured people so that they can learn from the experience of others. Hopefully this book will bring their accumulated experience to many other people.

I also want to recognize all of my friends at the Brain Injury Association of Minnesota, my professional second home. They are all a great source of support and knowledge and their tireless work on behalf of persons with brain injury is heroic. While I could list everyone there, those most helpful with this book in particular were Breanna Berthelsen, Brad Donaldson, and Pat Winnick.

I want to acknowledge all of the great colleagues at my practice who have blessed me with their friendship and hard work. In particular, I want to recognize Drs. Nancy Carlson and Tom Kern who have been with me for years. They are loyal, dedicated, intelligent—and a source of very pointed humor.

There are also other people who work diligently on behalf of persons with brain injury. These include two physicians who deserve recognition: Drs. Robert Sevenich and Kenneth Britton. Both are smart, insightful, and caring. They have always had my back. Also due for praise are Beth Bohnsack and Mike Sandmann, great colleagues and confidants.

Furthermore, I want to acknowledge the staff at Oxford for their faith in us. They believed in the value of this book when we proposed it and they helped us make it a much better book.

I owe an unpayable debt of gratitude to Patricia Florio, my second grade teacher at Longfellow Elementary School in Teaneck, NJ. She saved me.

In the real world outside of work, Bradley, Daniel, Hilleary, and Meredith are special people who care deeply about other people. They are just getting started in changing the world. Look out.

My brother Michael is a kind and gentle person. We are bound by shared experiences. He is special and I love him deeply.

My mother, Rhona, is the source of my compassion and I am in wonder at the sacrifices she made on my behalf. I have learned to cope with my grief at losing her.

Finally, Gwen. Nothing I achieve is complete without her, this book included. My work, my life, my self requires her.

—RLK

Contents

Introduction *3*

Lesson 1 Brain Injury Facts, Realities, and Inspirations *7*

Lesson 2 A New Sense of Self—Lost and Found *21*

Lesson 3 The Rehabilitation Hospital System: Staying Focused and Positive *37*

Lesson 4 Emotional Responses to Brain Injury—Reclaiming Grief *55*

Lesson 5 Anger, Guilt, Denial, and Behavior *71*

Lesson 6 Coping—How to Maintain a Healthy Outlook *99*

Lesson 7 Thoughts for People in the Lives of Those with Brain Injury *111*

Lesson 8 Getting Support *139*

Lesson 9 How to Keep on Recovering Well *159*

References *169*

About the Authors *179*

Index *183*

Therapists' Guide to Overcoming Grief and Loss After Brain Injury

Introduction

For professionals, helping people to cope after traumatic brain injury is particularly challenging. This injury is unique. Problems with self-awareness, a hallmark of brain injury, affect professionals' ability to address the complex emotional responses to brain injury and to engage and motivate people in treatment. Catastrophic reactions are possible when awareness begins to return prior to the healing brain's capacity for reasoning and problem-solving. Plus, for wounded warriors from two military campaigns who are returning in droves with blast and other types of brain injury, the situation is often complicated by stress reactions. Regardless of the circumstances of injury, it is common for unaware professionals to pathologize grief through clinical impression or psychometric tests. However, the bereavement literature suggests that many emotional reactions could be normal grief.

While good work is now underway to find the best ways to address the needs of persons with brain injury, scholars and researchers have a comparatively new interest in acquired brain injury. Articles began to be published just in the 1980s related to symptom description, epidemiology, and outcomes for traumatic brain injury, though stroke had been a focus in the scientific literature for a much longer time. Professionals have identified symptoms and established that this disorder usually causes multiple disabilities, with outcomes that get worse with increasing severity. Researchers are finding that the cognitive rehabilitation works, especially when delivered intensively and early in recovery. There has also been a great deal learned from persons with brain injury and from their caregivers and family members who have individually written accounts of their experiences.

Still, while there is more known now about the rehabilitation of acquired brain injury because of this research and work, many clinicians who wish to meet the emotional needs of people struggling to respond to the losses of this devastating injury, lack knowledge. This in turn leaves people with brain injury at a loss to find their emotional way.

Overcoming Grief and Loss After Brain Injury was written to address the needs of persons with brain injury and their families who seek the best interventions for facilitating positive and successful responses to the losses of brain injury. This book, *Therapists' Guide to Overcoming Grief and Loss After Brain Injury* is intended as a companion book to guide the professional helping persons with brain injury and their support system utilize the exercises in *Overcoming Grief and Loss After Brain Injury.*

The intent is for persons with brain injury or their support system to have a copy of *Overcoming Grief and Loss After Brain Injury.* The *Therapists' Guide* for the professional refers to exercises, handouts, figures, etc., in the companion book, but does not reproduce them. It is recommended that each person the professional is helping (person with brain injury, family member, etc.) have their own copy of the companion book so each can independently complete assignments. There is a Lesson specifically for those in the support system of persons with brain injury.

Though this book was informed by the current brain injury and bereavement literature, rather than being a scholarly work it is meant to be a practical resource. The exercises and information within the nine Lessons focus on helping people learn about the injury from a personal perspective. People are invited to relate each topic to their own injury experience, through questionnaires, exercises, and writing tasks.

The Lessons are organized in an order that illustrates a usual succession of concerns immediately following the injury and during later, post-acute periods. The person with a brain injury does not have to complete all of a Lesson at one time or for one session. Let them work at a pace they are comfortable with. Moreover, use your judgment as to what sequence you feel is best in which to present the Lessons. The Lessons appreciate that people will have a multitude of problems to address within each domain of concern. The intent is not to present an exhaustive list of treatments and interventions, but simply select the evidence-based methods for addressing specific cognitive, social, behavioral, and functional problems related to brain injury.

The rationale for the book includes the following concepts and literature-based beliefs about persons with brain injury.

- Persons with brain injury and family members will benefit from having information about brain injury and recovery.

- Persons with brain injury will be more motivated to participate fully in even challenging rehabilitation tasks if they understand the purpose of the tasks and their role in achieving successful recovery.

- If persons with brain injury have their range of emotions and thoughts normalized after injury they will be less likely to have stress or catastrophic reactions to changes in their skills and independence following injury.

- A comprehensive, informational book about adjustment after brain injury, which provides support and supported coping skill acquisition, will give them a head start in their recovery.

Goals of this book include the following:

- Provide a foundation of injury-related information about symptoms, normal emotional and behavioral disruptions, and coping skills

- Provide a structured, systematic, focused program of study

- Provide state-of-the-art treatment information related to enhancing outcomes for persons with brain injury

No book can address the myriad of issues and situations that can arise in clinical care, but we hope that we have provided you with processes and guideposts to facilitate your interventions.

Lesson 1   *Brain Injury Facts, Realities, and Inspirations*

Overview

The primary goal and intent of this Lesson is to assist clients with brain injury in identifying, understanding, and normalizing common symptoms and phases of recovery from brain injury. Lesson 1 clearly identifies causes of injury, symptoms that most people with brain injury and their family members report, and the purpose and substantive factors in acute- and post-acute rehabilitation. Using stories recounted by actual clients and family members touched by brain injury, you as therapist should use Lesson 1 to guide clients toward recognizing the best outlooks and approaches for avoiding pitfalls and enhancing the chances of a positive recovery.

Rationale

1. Persons with brain injury and their families have strong needs for information about brain injury symptoms and recovery.

2. Normalizing symptoms and recovery phases can be reassuring and prevent catastrophic reactions.

3. An understanding of the rehabilitation process and major players on most interdisciplinary teams will improve motivation and participation of clients with brain injury with regard to use of compensatory strategies or ongoing therapies.

4. Information about normal and pathological emotional reactions to brain injury will help clients and families more accurately

self-assess and more likely accept common ups and downs during recovery.

5. Personal stories involving survivors of brain injury will help the reader with brain injury identify with others who have this injury and will incentivize them and help them relate to the other material in the book.

6. The introduction of positive ideas and outlooks for coping will improve the hope, motivation, and effort of the person with brain injury during what is usually a life-long journey.

Presenting the Goals of This Lesson

Using the personal stories and examples provided in this and the companion book, the therapist can persuasively move persons with brain injury, and their family members, toward better post-injury adjustment through learning about common symptoms and causes of brain injury. Throughout the Lesson, the therapist should strive to supportively clarify post-injury symptoms, the purpose of rehabilitation, the members and roles of rehabilitation teams, and the importance of acceptance and use of strategies for successful recovery for their clients. The exercises and examples should be used to assist clients to identify, practice, and use outlooks and coping ideas that researchers, clinicians, and consumers tell us predict better long-term adjustment.

Review the following goals of this Lesson with clients.

- Learn about common causes and symptoms of brain injury
- Understand the stages of recovery from brain injury
- Learn about the major persons on your rehabilitation team
- Learn about the purpose of rehabilitation and your role in the process of getting better

Reassure clients that they will gain new understanding of the very common feelings and emotions they have been experiencing since their injury.

Begin by going over the comments reported by both clients and the rehabilitation providers who seek to support them in their recovery from brain injury. Be sure to emphasize that these are reported because they have been heard or said by so many people following a brain injury. Seek to educate clients about the enormity of the problem by pointing out that the direct quotes are from some of the millions of people each year in the United States who have brain injuries and experience loss of ability and independence as a result. Ask clients to turn to Box 1.1 in Lesson 1. in the companion book. Read each item aloud, allowing a few seconds for any client comments at the end of each quote.

Following collaborative review of the material in Box 1.1, and allowing plenty of time for clients to ask questions or provide some comments, mention that many of these persons went on to do well, with support and use of coping and other strategies.

Introduce a review of the causes of brain injury by either asking if clients will tell you how they got their brain injury, or, if you know this information, indicate that the cause of their injury is experienced by many other persons. Draw clients' attention to Box 1.2 in Lesson 1 of their book. Explain that this is a list of the most common causes of brain injury. Provide explanations of any causes that may be unclear or unknown for clients. Ask clients to notice that the cause of their brain injury is on the list, if that is known by now, and state how this makes it clear that they are not alone in their situation. If clients state that they do not know the cause of their brain injury, ask them to check with a family member, using the Box 1.2 list. Assure them, especially after they have identified the cause of their injury, that there are many in the larger community of persons around them with brain injury that have had similar experiences.

How About You?

Assist clients in identifying within themselves any of the feelings and concerns expressed by persons quoted in Box 1.1. If you are working with a caregiver or family member in addition to clients, ask the caregiver what possible feelings they think clients may be having that are similar to the quoted persons.

Assist clients in locating and completing the questionnaires (Boxes 1.3 to 1.5 in the companion book, Lesson 1) in the *How About You?* section. You may have to get permission from clients to ask someone who was with them at the time of the injury and knows the injury facts, if clients are not able to remember all of them. Having a caregiver present in the session would simplify the fact finding. Emphasize the reason for the questionnaires. Tell clients if they are more aware of the facts about their injury and the feelings they are having about it, they will find it easier to choose the best steps to take toward recovery. Assist clients by doing the writing if necessary. Make copies of their completed forms if they wish to take them home but suggest that all original materials be kept at the therapy setting to insure they will not get lost.

As always, allow some time for answering questions or listening to comments from clients.

Introduce the quotations in Box 1.6 in the companion book, Lesson 1, by talking about how the main character's struggles show how family members and significant others can also be touched by the losses associated with the injury.

Reassurance about "Invisible Symptoms"

Introduce the struggle with unawareness caused for persons with brain injury by the usual mismatch between the unchanged outward physical appearance and the mostly unseen cognitive and emotional changes related to the injury. Material in Box 1.7, found in Lesson 1 of the the companion book, as well as the story examples that follow, should be used to explain this conceptual frame clearly for clients. As always, accommodations should be made for the special learning needs of clients. You may have to select highlights from the materials to make the take-home points if clients have problems with reading and processing abstract or complex verbal, written information. The take-home points include:

1. Unseen or misunderstood symptoms of brain injury can lead to a damaging lack of awareness of deficits.

2. Problems with self-awareness, very common after brain injury, can impede return to former or similar vocational and interpersonal roles in the community for the recovering individual.

Introduce Brian's Story by stating that it contains examples of typical post-injury symptoms and struggles.

Brian's Story—A Success

Brian was driving home from an out-of-state business trip late one evening. The next thing he knew he was in a hospital bed with a headache. The strangers around him identified themselves as nurses or therapists. He had been in a serious motor vehicle accident and was in brain injury rehabilitation, he was told. He struggled to fight crushing fatigue, to organize his thoughts, think, and remember even a little of what had happened to him. He asked person after person, "Where am I?" "What happened to me?" When staff or relatives told him what happened, he found that he soon forgot what they had told him and had to ask again. He became irritated with those around him because they were having trouble understanding what he was saying for some reason. His family and the medical staff told him that a passing motorist had reported seeing his car in a gully. His car appeared to police to have drifted off the highway. He learned that his head struck the dashboard, resulting in a subarachnoid hemorrhage in the left side of his brain. Brian was determined to remember the cause of his accident. He asked everyone for clues but no one knew. He got a nurse to find a version of the police report in his medical chart admission papers. It was agonizingly short on details. "Male, 40's, status post single car crash, found with LOC (loss of consciousness) slumped forward on dash of his vehicle, 2:45 a.m. Left forehead laceration. Male transported to trauma center via medical rescue helicopter." As his thinking began to clear, Brian became aware of a weakness in his right hand and leg. He was annoyed as nurses and therapists told him not to get up without help, not to go to the bathroom without first calling them, that he couldn't have a drink of water until his swallowing test, and that he had to stay out of bed. When he tried to get up anyway, he was wobbly and had to grab furniture to avoid falling. One time he fell. Finding it hard to hide the frustration in their voices, the staff was constantly telling him not to get up or yelling, "Sit down!" At times Brian found himself wearing a cotton jacket that was tied to a chair so he couldn't get up. Staff would occasionally use soft arm bands to keep him restrained in his bed or chair, saying "it is to keep you safe." As he tried to ask questions or express his feelings and thoughts, he noticed that it was very hard to get his words to come out clearly. Brian's wife and son were overwhelmed, confused, embarrassed, and frustrated with him. Brian's wife and son treated him as if he were being rude or acting like a child. Though he could not figure out why, they seemed overwhelmed, confused, embarrassed, and frustrated by him. All Brian wanted to do was sleep, have people leave him alone, and find out what happened to him and why he didn't feel like himself anymore.

At this point in Brian's story, you should summarize issues with unawareness using the following points, with the goal of underscoring the potential for multiple problems caused by impaired self-awareness after brain injury.

- Brian's experience is quite common after a brain injury.
- Persons with brain injury often report they feel at first like they are in a fog.
- Fatigue is frequently a constant companion.
- Speech may be confused, slurred, and faint. It may be hard to understand the speech of others.
- The brain injury can cause a range of typical impairments in thinking skills, especially memory and reasoning.
- Persons with brain injury struggle to make sense out of their situation. They may feel restless, on an emotional roller coaster, and not as able to tolerate even minor frustrations. They can snap at those close to them.
- Persons with brain injury may be unsafe because they do not realize their limitations.
- Fear of loss of independence and control can drive people with brain injury to rebel against the staff and family who are trying to keep them safe.

Continue with Brian's story by stating that he was fortunate several forms of help became available for him as well as his family. State also that Brian's story shows a typical brain injury recovery path. Tell clients that Brian's story and the rest of the Lessons in this book will clarify how persons with brain injury and their family members are able to find and access healing and helpful resources. Provide the example that many people receive both inpatient and outpatient rehabilitation services following their brain injury.

Continue to review *Brian's Story* with clients, and call their attention to the positive outcomes.

Hope and Healing

Brian's initial inpatient rehabilitation was provided by a team of specialists including a physician, social worker, neuropsychologist, physical therapist, speech language pathologist, occupational therapist, recreational therapist, and nurse specialist. He was given medication temporarily to help him sleep better at night and stay awake and alert during the day therapies. He made excellent progress with his walking and was able to leave the hospital with only a cane for assistance for balance. His rehabilitation program included a number of different therapies as well as education. He spent at least one, and sometimes two sessions a day with the neuropsychologist, social worker, occupational therapist, and speech therapist learning about his injury as well as practicing memory and thinking strategies. The team of therapists also trained him to monitor and control his behavior consistently so he could be less impulsive, as well as safe and appropriate with others. Counseling was helping him, and his family, understand and accept the challenges resulting from his brain injury. His characteristic kind and caring ways were slowly returning to his daily interactions with family and friends.

Brian was fortunate to also receive outpatient rehabilitation. Many people, like Brian, transfer from inpatient to outpatient rehabilitation in a fairly short period of time—two weeks to one month. Like Brian, they make progress in inpatient brain injury rehabilitation, but may still have some problems to work on. Outpatient therapy teams usually do a new assessment or evaluation of the person with the brain injury. They often have a report from the inpatient team. So the outpatient therapists compare their new evaluation findings with the old report to get an accurate picture of clients' current skills and abilities. The outpatient team then set new goals based on the new evaluation because these new goals can then reflect the next step in recovery. Over the next 12 months, a typical time frame for most persons following discharge from an inpatient brain injury unit, Brian's outpatient rehabilitation therapists began to get him ready to resume work. He was able to obtain a job through his state's department of rehabilitation services. A job "coach" went to work with him for a while to help problem solve any barriers to Brian's becoming a productive worker. With family support, Brian has managed to regain much of what he lost and is successfully relying on new ideas for coping.

Brian's story is a good illustration of what many people with brain injury experience during their initial recovery time, the first several months after injury.

Now direct clients' attention to Box 1.8 in Lesson 1 of their books. Introduce the information as a helpful summary of the activities and major professionals in brain injury rehabilitation. The "Rehabilitation Team Members and Their Jobs" information will help introduce the rehabilitation process and major players to clients. Even if clients attended both acute- and post-acute rehabilitation many months ago, the information may clarify the purpose of that process for them and hopefully renew their efforts to draw upon skills and knowledge acquired during that time. This will be especially true if they were experiencing more severe levels of impaired self-awareness during their rehabilitation. The information in Box 1.8 is an overview of the rehabilitation process and major players. Point out that later on in your work together, Lesson 3, "The Rehabilitation Hospital System: Staying Focused and Positive," will provide clients with more detailed information and concepts about rehabilitation.

You should clearly explain the instructions for using the activity in Box 1.8 to clients. Emphasize that understanding the purpose and reasons for rehabilitation allows persons with brain injury to participate more fully and get the most out of their hard work in therapies. If rehabilitation has been completed, it can help reinforce the need to use strategies and information gained during those experiences to help improve functioning.

Following completion of the activity in Box 1.8, you should help clients try to recall and talk about their rehabilitation experiences. After guiding clients in discussing their best and not so great experiences, talk with them about any gaps they may have had during their rehabilitation. Explore with them how this may have made a difference, or explain what that portion of their rehabilitation would have been focused on. As a result of this exercise, clients may report that they did not experience all of the modalities or team members listed in Box 1.8 at the time of their rehabilitation. They may express regret or a wish to obtain such services and a vision of how that would be helpful now. You can then assist clients in making a connection with available community resources that are within their means. You can also use this as an avenue to begin providing appropriate cognitive behavior therapy and rehabilitation as a part of your work with them.

The following stories should now be reviewed with clients to illustrate the difficulties persons with brain injury may encounter when they are not able to obtain rehabilitation services. The goals are to point out the value of such services and instill motivation in clients to use all information and strategies they were taught in rehabilitation or to shore up their determination to participate fully in current and ongoing therapies. You should ask clients, after each story, what they thought of the events and people involved. It will also be important to ask clients what they think Pat, Audrey, their children, or John were feeling and how they were coping with their situations. Finally, you should ask whether clients had similar experiences and feelings.

Introduce the story below as an example of the value of rehabilitation after brain injury.

Pat's Story—Challenges and Despair

Not every person with brain injury is able to have rehabilitation. In addition to financial reasons, an incorrect diagnosis, that totally misses the existence of a brain injury, can occur. Let look at the following story to see how a brain injury can go undiscovered with drastic consequences.

After seven months, Pat finally made an appointment to take her three children to see a therapist. She needed help with parenting. Since her car accident almost one year ago, family life had become chaotic. Everyday chores seemed overwhelming to Pat. Her ability to manage had been dwindling and she was losing her temper more and more frequently with the kids. She couldn't get the 6-year-old to sleep in her own bed. The 10- and 13-year-olds were fighting with each other and baiting the youngest until she cried. They all refused to do what she asked them to do. Her husband was also recovering from neck, back, and leg injuries, so could not manage them well either.

Pat's return to work, eight months after the accident, brought the behavioral and parenting challenges at home to a crisis point. With the advice of a friend Pat made an appointment with a local family therapist. The psychologist took one look at the waiting room full of out-of-control children, the passive and bewildered mother, and asked Pat to come in first. During the interview, the psychologist began to ask a lot of questions about the accident. Pat reported what doctors, nurses, and family members told her, explaining to the psychologist that she herself could not really recall a thing. She and her husband were coming home from a wonderful New Year's Eve dinner at a local restaurant when their car was hit broadside by a pizza delivery truck. As a result of the impact, her husband's right shoulder pushed into her left chest, breaking eight of her ribs and collapsing a lung. Both of them were feared near death. They had to be cut out of their car and were rushed to a local hospital trauma center.

Doctors in the emergency room quickly sent Pat up to the Operating Room where surgeons worked to re-inflate her lung and remove her spleen. The final physician's summary stated that most of the couples' injuries were in their chest and extremities and that they would eventually recover. Family members took care of the children for the three weeks that she and her husband were in the hospital and for the two months they were ambulating with crutches at home. Pat and her husband were in pain and on various pain medications for a long time. The youngest child was tearful, anxious, and clingy. She refused to sleep in her own bed.

Pat was very happy to return to work. However, Pat, once known for her organization and time management in running a busy household of five and holding down a demanding managerial job, did not seem to have any energy or skills anymore. Details began to slip through her fingers. Major mistakes became frequent, both at the office and at home. Dinner did not seem to get on the table regularly. The children were not getting to bed on time. All her husband wanted to do was take his pain medication and sleep. He had applied for and received disability insurance and was not able to return to work.

After talking with Pat and administering some cognitive tests, the psychologist finally met with all of them. She referred Pat to a neurologist, reporting to Pat that the test results suggested that the accident may have caused a brain injury, perhaps not known or diagnosed at the time. Pat and her children were told about brain injury symptoms and given printed information from the Brain Injury Association of America (www.biausa.org). As it turned out, Pat was later diagnosed with a moderately severe anoxic brain injury caused by a lack of oxygen to her brain at the time of the accident. She was referred for and went through outpatient rehabilitation. She learned strategies for coping with her memory problems and was able to resume her job on a part-time basis. She improved her parenting skills, though she required parenting help with and counseling for her children. Fortunately her family had the financial resources to provide the help she needed.

Introduce *Audrey and John's Story* and tell clients that it will help them understand a family member's perspective after brain injury.

Audrey and John's Story

At 5 p.m. Audrey knew her husband was nearing home after one of his truck runs up the coast. Tonight she did not receive his usual CB-radio call telling her he was almost there. Instead a highway patrolman arrived to tell her John had been taken to a hospital about one hour away. She threw on her coat, called her mother to come watch their 6-year-old twins, and took off for the emergency room.

Audrey heard from the emergency room staff that a passing motorist notified police that John was driving slowly and weaving all over the road. John actually was able to radio his company dispatcher to tell her he was feeling sick, pull his truck over, and put on the brake, before collapsing on the steering wheel. Hospital staff worked to stabilize John. A scan revealed an aneurysm, a small "bubble" of one of the blood vessels in his brain, had burst. A team of surgeons operated to drain the blood, removing a piece of his skull to prevent further damage from swelling. Audrey was overjoyed to see her husband when they finally took John back to his room in Neuroscience Intensive Care. The helmet covering the exposed portion of his head was a constant reminder of how close a call this was.

John was quiet for a few days, receiving nutrition and medicine from tubes and IVs. Then he started to move restlessly. He would open his eyes when Audrey called his name but close them again quickly. "Does he still know me?" Audrey wondered. John's days and nights were mixed up. He was up at night and wanted to sleep during the day. The few words he spoke were scrambled or mixed up. Despite being told to leave his helmet on, he kept trying to take it off. He pulled out his IV twice. Audrey missed her twins but tried to stay with John at night, while her mother was at home with the children. She was exhausted during the day, trying to keep up with her sons. John was embarrassing her. He tried to grab the nurses and ask them for kisses. He was demanding and ungrateful toward Audrey. He pleaded for her to take him home and became enraged when she said she could not.

John's progress was slow, and he was moved to a nursing home for a time. His behavior improved, but he still acted like a child much of the time. Audrey was able to be home with her children more, but she missed her partner and spouse. Finances nearing collapse, Audrey took a part-time job. She was forced to learn about the banking and finances, and struggled to find out what she could about community resources for her husband's return. She fought her own depression, especially when friends and relatives told her "You should be grateful he survived!" It was difficult for her to be the loving, helpful wife when this man she married now seemed like a stranger.

Summary

Point out for clients that the two stories above are about real persons and their families and recur often on the typical brain injury rehabilitation unit or outpatient mental health clinic. Clients should also be told that the symptoms displayed, the feelings, the struggles, and the losses experienced by Audrey, John, Pat, and their families are common markers of the beginning of the life-long journey of persons who have sustained brain injuries and their family members. You should reassure clients by explaining that Lesson 1 has revealed how many people share these same, common, and normal responses to brain injury. The large number of persons with brain injury in their community and in the United States provides a network of support for clients and has helped doctors and providers learn about this injury. Armed with knowledge from their study of these common symptoms and problems, therapists are now better able to give clients and others the training and information they need to continue a successful recovery.

Lesson 2   *A New Sense of Self—Lost and Found*

Overview

The purpose of Lesson 2 is to provide persons with brain injury and their family members and caregivers with evidence-based compensatory strategies and coping methods to help them work through grief about post-injury losses and changes and adjust more successfully. Using the material and exercises in Lesson 2, therapists can help their clients with brain injury identify common post-injury symptoms and more accurately define their range of problems with cognition, fatigue, executive functions, and social behavior. For example, among the many deficits that clients and family members report following brain injury, behavioral and communication difficulties may be among the most limiting and socially isolating. Lesson 2 focuses on giving clients specific tools for overcoming post-injury cognitive, physical, functional, social and behavioral challenges through descriptions, aids to self-understanding of deficits, and guided practice of techniques that bolster skills in these important domains of post-injury concern. The ideas presented are an overview of methods, each of which could take weeks to present and learn. Clients' ability to learn and apply the techniques will be enhanced by assistance from a therapist knowledgeable and experienced in implementing evidence-based compensatory cognitive and coping interventions and training. Prior reading from the References provided at the end of this book will refresh your acquaintance with evidence-based neurobehavioral interventions for persons with brain injury. In addition, the likelihood of successful intervention and training will be exponentially increased if you are able to see results of prior neuropsychological and neurobehavioral testing prior to beginning work with clients. Matching of clients' unique deficits and strength profiles with the strategies that are most relevant for them is strongly recommended. Your selection of interventions most suited to clients' needs should also be informed by your awareness of their level of ability—that is, the degree to which they are dependent on external cues to consistently use compensatory or metacognitive strategies.

Rationale

1. Persons with brain injury and their families will feel more confident and in control of their own recovery if they possess a number of evidence-based coping tools and strategies for overcoming injury-related deficits.

2. The grief about injury-related losses that most persons with brain injury experience can be made more tolerable when there is active and consistent effort to use and benefit from compensatory and coping strategies.

3. Persons with brain injury and their families who understand and can practice self-management of common brain injury symptoms will enjoy more satisfying interpersonal relationships, and be more employable.

4. An understanding of the complexity and nuances of social communication will help the person with brain injury have a better quality of life.

5. Personal stories involving survivors of brain injury will help the reader with brain injury identify with others who have this injury and will incentivize them and help them relate to the other material in the book.

6. Tools for improving the common cognitive, physical, and emotional challenges of brain injury will build confidence and competence in the person with brain injury.

Presenting the Goals of This Lesson

Review the following goals for the Lesson with clients.

- Identify common post-brain-injury challenges
- Identify the client's specific challenges
- Learn strategies for managing post-injury physical problems
- Learn strategies for managing post-injury impairments of attention, memory, problem-solving, self-management of behavior, emotions and coping, and communication

Tell clients that persons with brain injury often say "I just don't feel like myself." They describe it as a strange feeling, a loss, and have trouble putting it into words. Many times this new sense of self does not go away. Ask clients if they have had that odd sense of being different than they were before their injury. If they acknowledge this feeling, reassure them that they are fortunate because brain injury experts actually know a lot about common symptoms of brain injury that are often the cause of that different sensation. Even if your clients with brain injury do not report awareness of feeling different, you can serve as a reassuring guide in helping them identify some of their more troublesome but common post-injury symptoms and teaching them effective coping strategies.

Explain to clients that not knowing how the brain injury affected them can make it hard for them to know what to do to feel more like themselves and on top of things again. Tell them that knowing will reassure them that they are experiencing normal symptoms for a person with a brain injury and will also allow them to take advantage of strategies and coping methods that can best help them progress in recovery. Explain that adjustment to these symptoms and changes after injury will improve their coping with grief and make the feelings more tolerable because they will be actively participating in improving their situation.

Explain that no two people are alike and that every brain injury is therefore completely unique. People get better at different rates. Some people have mild brain injuries, while others have severe injuries. The biggest post-injury loss many face is poor balance and other physical changes. Others struggle with speech and memory problems. When a person goes from good physical health to experiencing physical, language, and memory problems, the transition is accompanied by the emotions of loss and grief. Introduce some examples to illustrate these issues.

Tim's Story

Tim fell off a roof when he was installing gutters and had a brain injury. Doctors told him that he made a good physical recovery and he was discharged from the hospital. Tim still feels tired most of the time, and barely has enough energy to get up, have breakfast, and watch television. He wonders why he is so tired. He worries that something is terribly wrong with him.

Jason's Story

At the garage where he is employed full time as a mechanic, a small part on a car engine broke off while Jason was testing the new sparkplugs he had installed. When his co-worker started the engine, the metal part went flying and into the front of Jason's skull, then his brain. Jason did not lose consciousness. He was discharged and sent home quickly from the hospital after his injury and the surgery to remove the metal piece. Jason's vision was blurry though, and he is still having trouble seeing. The sunlight makes it harder for him to see. He is worried about being able to go back to work.

Jane's Story

Jane was in a car crash. She didn't remember anything until she woke up in the hospital. It bothers her not to remember. She works as a waitress and she thinks she might have trouble remembering all the customers' orders. She is also having trouble sleeping at night. Jane worries that she is going crazy.

Tell clients that fatigue, blurred or impaired vision, and memory problems are very common after brain injury but, unfortunately, no one told Tim, Jason, and Jane about typical brain injury symptoms and they began to feel hopeless and afraid. Point out that Tim was sad about losing energy and endurance, Jason about his loss of vision, and Jane about her loss of memory. Tell clients if they are experiencing any of these symptoms, they are likely grieving as well and may find the ideas for improvement in Lesson 2 helpful.

How About You? How Are You Doing?

Direct clients to the "Brain Injury Symptom Questionnaire" (BISQ) in Box 2.1, in Lesson 2 of their books. Explain that it can help them identify any common post-injury symptoms they may be experiencing. Tell them to check all items that are true, and to be as honest as possible. If they are not sure, ask them if others have noticed and told them that they have the symptom. Tell clients that the questionnaire is long because there are a large number of people with brain injury symptoms and that they report many different kinds of symptoms in a range of combinations. Tell them that as they read through the questionnaire, they should notice that their symptoms are not as unusual as they may have thought. Tell clients that the list can be divided into three sections that represent three parts of recovery from a brain injury. Explain that recovery from brain injury is part physical (P), part cognitive (C), and part emotional and behavioral (EB) and that the letters by the check boxes on the list show which type of symptom each item is. Explain further that the divisions in the Questionnaire helps group the ideas for improving according to type of symptom.

Ask clients to notice how many symptoms they checked. Ask also whether they checked more P symptoms, or C symptoms, or EB symptoms—or a mixture of all three? Note that everyone is different, with different challenges in different symptom areas. Explain that identification of their own unique set of symptoms is a very important starting place. Once they know what they need to work on they can choose the right strategies and ideas for recovery. The therapist should call clients' attention to the letters in parentheses next to the information and strategy sections below so that they can refer back to their Box 2.1, Lesson 2 questionnaire responses and match their symptoms to the ideas offered for improvement of each item they endorsed.

Improving Post-Injury Physical Symptoms (P)

Fatigue and Restlessness

Tell clients that people with brain injury fall into three groups related to sleep and restlessness.

1. Some feel tired all the time. They may have drowsy periods during the day, even after a full night's sleep. They complain about always feeling tired.

2. Others are very restless and have trouble sitting still. Staff and family members tell them to "slow down" or "wait for help before you get up."

3. Still other people with brain injury are a combination of both kinds; they feel tired during the day because they have trouble sleeping at night.

Tell clients that they may identify with one of these groups.

Direct clients' attention to the "Coping with Fatigue and Restlessness After Brain Injury" in Box 2.2, Lesson 2 of their books. Introduce it by stating that there are several causes and helps for sleepiness, sleeplessness, and restlessness. Note that the table contains ways of looking first at the causes of and then the ideas for improvement of sleep and energy problems after brain injury. Explain that Box 2.2 shows several reasons for disturbed sleep and energy.

- First, explain to clients that the actual neurological injury and resulting changes in the brain are part of the reason that people have difficulty with either sleep or restlessness afterward. Since there are actual changes in the chemistry and structure of the brain from the injury, medications often work well to help with this.

Explain that a physician who is aware of the needs of clients with brain injury will know best whether medication will help them, and what type they need, for how long. Explain also that challenges with sleep and restlessness usually get better over time.

- Second, people often have pain due to headache or injuries to their bodies that they sustain during their accident. The pain can keep them up at night, which results in drowsiness during the day. Tell clients that the brain injury physician is experienced in choosing a pain medication that will reduce discomfort without making a person drowsy. Be sure to emphasize for clients the importance of reporting their pain and taking any medication prescribed as instructed. Add that as all injuries heal, the pain will most likely get less intense.

- A third cause of sleep/restlessness problems can be the medications themselves. Explain that some medications that are needed for behavior or pain can also have behavioral and arousal side effects. State that the best choice in dealing with sleepiness due to medication is to ask their doctor if there is a different dosing pattern than can help. Provide an example as follows: If they normally take their medication in the morning, and think it makes them sleepy, they should ask their doctor if they can take it at night or split the dose, taking half in the morning and half in the evening. They certainly want to be sleepy at night!

- Fourth, explain that worry can interfere with sleep and behavior. There are many realities to deal with after a brain injury. Bills are still coming in. They may worry about getting back to work to support themselves. They may worry about their bills. Tell clients that worry actually does little good. Explain that there are options and solutions for crises involving housing, finances, family issues, and getting back to work. Social workers are members of rehabilitation teams and community service centers that provide help with this. Furthermore, explain that other Lessons in the book will provide more information about getting emotional supports as well as many links and information about community-based aids for adjustment and return to work.

You should next introduce the "3-Minute Chill-Out Technique," in Box 2.3, Lesson 2 of the companion book, explaining that it is a technique for relaxing to improve their ability to manage restlessness or sleep restfully, even while they continue working out all these post-injury challenges and issues day to day. As you demonstrate each step, be sure to do each along with clients.

- Explain that a fifth cause of sleeplessness and restlessness can be diet. Encourage clients to make good dietary and nutritional choices, and avoid highly caffeinated drinks and foods not part of a special diet they may require to maintain good health, such as a diabetic diet.

Balance and Dizziness

Tell clients that problems with balance and dizziness can result in falls and additional injury, which can result in lengthening recovery time after brain injury. Explain that in the typical inpatient or outpatient rehabilitation center, it is usually the physical therapist who works with persons who have balance problems after brain injury. Persons with brain injury will get the most benefit from physical therapy for balance problems if they try their best to come to therapies on time and work as hard as they can, even if they are tired or have some discomfort. Dizziness can be caused by the injury itself, visual disturbances, inner ear problems, and can cause nausea and distraction. Explain that physicians can often help, if needed, with medication changes, an eye patch, or by recommending increased rest breaks to improve dizziness and reduce risk of falls. Explain that certain behavioral strategies will also help, including slowing down when moving around, taking time to get up from a sitting position, and trying not to get distracted when moving around. If the client has balance or dizziness issues, encourage them to focus on moving, rather than talking, watching television, or trying to look at something out the window.

Lower and Upper Body Weakness and Gait Problems

Explain to clients that just as with balance and dizziness, steady work on all the exercises and activities planned by their physical therapist (PT) will improve their lower body strength and gait. The PT will know how much should be done, how soon, and how fast. In addition, tell clients that the occupational therapist (OT) is usually the rehabilitation team member who provides therapy to strengthen the upper body. The OTs also help clients with brain injury to practice daily activities like dressing, grooming, and work-related tasks.

Improving Post-Injury Cognitive Impairments (C)

Confusion

Tell clients that confusion is usually seen as an early brain injury symptom, but can also occur if the person with the brain injury is tired or having to deal with more than one task or difficulty at a time. Recommend consistent use of compensatory aids for memory like calendars, schedules, a dry erase board with daily information, and a memory log for keeping them on top of daily facts. Explain that caregivers can help by calling the person's attention to these environmental aids, or assisting in their consistent use of memory aids. Posting all of the aids in highly visible places is also a big help. Tell clients that family members and friends can provide verbal reminders, or cues, until clients become independent and consistent with their use of the aids. When confusion continues to be a problem, encourage clients to contact their brain injury physician who can recommend some medications that are known to improve this. Introduce the "Daily Information Sheet" in Box 2.4, Lesson 2 of the companion book, stating that it is designed to be used consistently every day. Show clients how to transfer the sheet to a dry erase board so entries can be erased and the board space reused many times without waste of paper. Explain that consistent use of the sheet over time will help reduce confusion.

Problems with Attention/Concentration

Tell clients that distractibility is a frequent problem after brain injury. Ask if clients have noticed that they have difficulty focusing or concentrating. Tell them that poor concentration is a frustrating brain injury symptom for a number of reasons. People need to be able to pay attention to be safe, learn, remember, follow instructions vital to recovery, manage money, and do daily tasks. Review the strategies in Box 2.5, Lesson 2 of the companion book, introducing them as helpful ideas for improving attention.

Memory

This section on memory is an excellent opportunity for therapists to give clients an in-depth grasp of one of the most challenging and universal post-injury deficits. Using a positive approach, therapists should review with clients that there are several kinds of memory, with particular attention to short term, delayed, long term, and prospective as those most frequently addressed by rehabilitation providers. Tell them the good news is that most people keep long-term recall following brain injury. As examples, ask clients if they remember their mother's name, address if they have lived in the same place for many years, or the name of the last school they went to. This is a good example because most people can quickly retrieve and say this information. Therapists should then explain that remembering new information, like names of people you have not known very long, is more difficult after brain injury. Problems with delayed memory and prospective memory can disrupt their daily routine and work. Explain that delayed memory refers to the ability to recall what happened, what you read, what you heard, and what you saw several minutes to hours later. Tell them that prospective memory is being able to remember to follow through with something you scheduled or planned for at an earlier time. It is frustrating to forget information, and sometimes dangerous! Boxes 2.6 and 2.7 of Lesson 2 in the companion book contain evidence-based ideas for compensating for deficits in both these types of memory. Assist clients in reading and trying out the multiple strategies. Demonstrate the NAME mnemonic and other strategies, taking extra time if necessary, to be sure that clients have really mastered the steps and see the value. Assignment and review of between-session practice of specific strategies, depending on the particular memory deficits you have identified for each individual client, are recommended.

Problem Solving

This section on problem solving moves toward the domain of executive functioning, which involves several areas often impaired following brain injury—reasoning, self-awareness, self-management, memory, attention. Clients need to have all of these abilities available to them in an integrated way for success in accomplishing day-to-day tasks as well as vocational and avocational initiatives. Unfortunately, these cognitive abilities are usually diminished as a result of the brain injury, in varying degrees of severity. You can help clients in two ways with improving their executive functioning skills with Lesson 2 content. First, you can increase clients' understanding of the complexity of the area and, second, you can teach and encourage consistent use of strategies for improvement.

Start by explaining that clients can have several possible challenges to problem solving after a brain injury. Clients should be told that some very important cognitive abilities used in problem solving, such as memory, attention, and decision making, are often impaired when someone experiences a brain injury. Tell clients that, in addition, people often have more difficulty with generating or thinking of more than one solution to a problem after brain injury. Introduce the SOLVE strategy in Box 2.8, Lesson 2 of the companion book. Tell them that this is a mnemonic strategy that can help them make the process of problem solving easier and more productive. Tell clients that the SOLVE strategy is like the NAME strategy for memory that was described earlier, in that each letter stands for a step in the strategy. Recommend that they consistently use this step-wise, clear approach to improving their ability to effectively solve problems.

Provide the example in Box 2.9 in Lesson 2 of the companion book as a way of demonstrating how this strategy can work for clients.

Now assist clients to practice more on their own. Encourage them to provide a real problem to try out further use of the S-O-L-V-E strategy. Have extra copies of the format or write the headings on several copies of paper to help the client practice with your support and guidance.

Improving Post-Injury Emotional, Social, and Behavioral Problems with Recovery Strategies (EB)

This section of Lesson 2 will allow therapists to assist clients in addressing any emotional, social, and behavioral skill areas that can be disrupted after brain injury. Therapists will first present a social and behavioral challenge, then present ideas for improving and coping. The areas addressed will be executive, emotional, and social functioning. You can present both information about common post-injury problems with emotional and social functioning and strategies for emotional and behavioral self-management, as well as ideas for finding and maintaining satisfying relationships.

Executive Functioning: Behavioral Self-management

Explain to clients that after brain injury many people have difficulty with self-awareness and self-regulation. As a result, friends and caregivers may see them as unsafe, and tell to "slow down" or watch them closely. Friends and family may be insulted when the person with the brain injury blurts out inappropriate comments without thinking. Tell clients that people with brain injury may find this unwanted supervision or reactions to their behavior very irritating because they are adults and want to be independent, but do not realize that they are acting in an unsafe or rude manner. Unfortunately, the brain injury often changes what is safe for the person to do, and the person may not yet have healed enough to be aware of this. Tell clients that it can take a fall, and further injuries, for the person with the brain injury to realize that things are different. Encourage clients to avoid taking chances with risky or socially inappropriate actions and improve self-management with purposeful use of the "Be Your Own Coach" (BYOC) Strategy. Introduce the strategy by commenting that everyone has had or has been a coach at one time or another in their lives. Ask clients to tell you what the main jobs of a coach are. If they say either "tell the players what to do," or "say positive and encouraging things to the players," tell them they are correct. If they do not mention these answers, provide them for clients by writing them down with the heading "Jobs of a Coach." Explain that the BYOC strategy is very simple. If they function as their own coach, and use the strategy, they will tell themselves what to do—before they do it, and talk to themselves in positive ways. Introduce the story below, reading it to clients if needed, as an example.

Jim's Story

Jim was serving as pitcher in a baseball game and took a line drive to his head. He was unconscious and later testing at the hospital revealed a brain injury. While Jim recovered in the hospital, his family and therapists noticed he was very impulsive. His parents watched him like a hawk. They made him mad because they followed him around, even to the bathroom! They just thought he was moving too quickly and were worried. Jim got fed up and had some heated arguments with his parents. The family was referred to a neuropsychologist who showed Jim how to coach himself, to tell himself "Stop, think, plan" every time he got ready to do something. This self-coaching gave Jim a few seconds more, a few seconds to avoid jumping up so quickly that he fell or tripped. In time Jim's parents trusted him to function alone as his control of himself improved using the BYOC strategy. They relaxed as Jim began to more safely take charge of his own life again.

Talk with clients about some situations where, if they had used the BYOC strategy, they might have avoided unpleasant consequences. Encourage clients to use the strategy and let you know how it is working for them.

Improving Social and Emotional Functioning

Explain to clients that, after brain injury, many people tend to blurt out inappropriate or rude comments, get too personal with questions and remarks, and have problems with remembering facts that are important for keeping a relationship going. Explain that any or all of these problems can put some distance between them and the people they care about or the people they would like to meet and get to know. Tell clients that they may find that is it also more difficult to manage strong feelings since their injury. Having angry or tearful outbursts can also put a strain on relationships. Tell them, in a nutshell, self-control, memory, and communication, which can all be more difficult for the person with a brain injury, are very important ingredients in getting along well with others. Recommend the BYOC strategy again and tell clients that it can help maintain the kind of self-control needed for all types of relationships. In addition, getting help from a physician who is experienced with treating people with brain injury can help in terms of getting medication for controlling intense feelings and behavior problems. Direct clients to reread the sections of Lesson 1 related to coping with post-injury emotional ups and downs. Tell them that there are many helpful ideas and discussions in this Lesson, as well as in Lesson 4 ahead, about feelings following brain injury and how to cope successfully with these. Explain that having emotional ups and downs is normal after brain injury. Positive self-talk and motivation to achieve doable goals are ways to reduce the intensity of the lows.

Remembering the Important Things for Relationships

Remind clients of the multiple ideas discussed above for improving memory and tell them that all can be applied to improve relationships with friends and family. Provide the example of a possible worry that they might forget a friend or family member's birthday, or an anniversary. Suggest combining the two strategies of using a calendar and writing things down. They can write important dates on their calendar and place it in a very visible place. As they turn the calendar pages, with the passage of months, they will be reminded by their own notes! Suggest the SOLVE strategy for working out conflict with others in a productive manner, something that can be difficult after brain injury. Explain that if they work together with their friend, family member, or partner, and use the SOLVE strategy described earlier in this Lesson, they may reduce conflict and make progress toward improving their relationships. Using extra practice sheets, follow the strategy with an interpersonal example such as: you want your friend to go to the movies with you but he or she is tired and want to stay home.

Effective Communication

Explain that brain injury often makes clear communication a challenge. There are problems with being understood by others, understanding what others say, keeping up with the topic in a fast moving group conversation, talking too much or too little, and with listening to others without interrupting. Introduce the ideas for improving communication presented in Box 2.10 by explaining that communication between people involves talking, listening, and nonverbal communication. Tell them that Box 2.10, Lesson 2 of the companion book suggests ideas for improving each of these parts of communication in order to improve relationships and interactions with others. Read through all of the ideas with clients, demonstrating with role plays, so they can practice these techniques and suggestions. Encourage consistent use of the guidelines and ask them to let you know how these are working during their interactions with others.

Summary

Review the many concepts and strategies covered in Lesson 2. Explain that the information and ideas will guide them to look closely at their post-injury self, and take stock of all the strengths and weaknesses that will go with them as they continue to get better. Explain that while loss is a part of brain injury, they will be ahead of the game by being able to clearly identify what they have lost. Tell them that at first this may not make sense. They might think "I feel sad and angry about losing my ability to speak clearly." However, explain that their grief about their losses can be more tolerable if they actively use coping ideas to overcome what is now more difficult for them to do. Tell them that they should also take comfort in the strengths they still have.

If they realize their remaining strengths, they can benefit more from therapies and conscious, consistent use of coping strategies. Point out that use of the tools and ideas in Lesson 2 will help move them through their grief and toward a more satisfying, independent, and less stressful post-injury life.

Lesson 3

The Rehabilitation Hospital System: Staying Focused and Positive

Overview

The preceding lessons introduced the idea that challenges are a normal part of coping after brain injury and that there are concrete strategies persons with brain injury can use to make life easier. For many persons with brain injury, the coping process begins during rehabilitation. This Lesson addresses how persons with brain injury can be most successful during the time in the hospital. However, if you are helping people who never went to a rehabilitation hospital or have already left, you can adapt relevant parts of this Lesson to assist them to better understand the health care players they may still encounter, or want to seek out, in a clinic situation and how they function.

The goal of this Lesson is to facilitate the rehabilitation experience for persons with brain injury. In doing so, you can enhance the treatment experience, decreasing later sense of loss by enhancing early therapeutic success. The major ideas that you will want to teach in this Lesson are:

1. How the rehabilitation system works
2. How rehabilitation differs from other health care
3. What role the person with brain injury has in rehabilitation

Parts of this Lesson address the role of psychologists. If you are a psychologist, then you can use that part of this Lesson to introduce your own role. However, the Lesson is written assuming another professional is explaining the role psychologists play on the team since diverse therapists may be using this guide with persons with brain injury.

Rationale

1. Too often persons with brain injury fail to obtain the maximum benefit they might receive from rehabilitation because of lack of preparedness. The grief and sense of loss persons with brain injury experience can be reduced through maximizing the success of rehabilitation.

2. Persons with brain injury can be frustrated when they are unprepared for a focus on improvement and compensation, not cure. In acute care they are often told that things will be fine, which they take to mean as "normal," but in rehabilitation the emphasis on advancement and accommodation requires a different mindset. Persons with brain injury are typically ill prepared for this switch.

3. Rehabilitation takes hard work on the part of the persons with brain injury, whereas in acute care the persons with brain injury may have been a passive recipient of care. Once again, the demands of rehabilitation can be stressful for persons with brain injury when their expectations are based on their acute-care experiences.

4. In rehabilitation, time is spent working on deficits, things that the persons with brain injury are not doing well, whereas in real life people spend their time on things they do well (e.g., jobs, hobbies, social activities) and try to avoid areas of weakness. Hence, rehabilitation can be unpleasant since therapy is hard work. In the real world people spend their day working at tasks they have good skills for; in rehabilitation the persons with brain injury spend their days in therapy working at the skills they are struggling with. Readiness for this can help them tolerate rehabilitation better.

5. Seeking emotional help needs normalizing because rehabilitation can be emotionally challenging.

6. Knowing how to communicate needs and preferences during rehabilitation is essential to interface with the rehabilitation team and achieve maximum satisfaction during rehabilitation.

7. Some treatment (e.g., cognitive rehabilitation exercises) during therapy may lack face validity. Awareness of the nature of treatment can ease acceptance and participation in treatment.

8. Knowing how to conceptualize treatment termination is helpful for self-esteem and taking the next steps.

9. Families can have issues with their role in facilitating rehabilitation, as persons with brain injury need to be prepared for their family's responses, which is essential for optimum outcome.

Presenting the Goals of This Lesson

The central idea to convey in readying the persons with brain injury for this Lesson is that rehabilitation is different than previous life experiences and different from past acute health care, but with a little help they can easily navigate rehabilitation. If they view it as if it is a cross-cultural experience in which there are different roles and rules to understand, then they will feel more comfortable learning the system and getting the most out of rehabilitation. You can provide them reassurance that you will teach them the "customs" of rehabilitation.

Review the following goals for the Lesson with clients.

- To better understand the rehabilitation hospital system
- To learn the differences between traditional and rehabilitation care
- To be more comfortable during rehabilitation
- To understand their family's response to their rehabilitation

Addressing Common Responses to Rehabilitation

They may be thinking that they are the only ones who find rehabilitation unusual and stressful. Check with them to see if any of following statements are similar to thoughts that they have been having.

- "This is so different from the acute hospital unit."

- "My surgeon said I was going to be fine, but here they keep discussing compensating for deficits."

- "My therapists are talking about discharge, but I don't feel ready."

- "I don't know why they want me to see a psychologist."

- "As a family member, I feel lost; everyone is focused on my loved one, but I have worries, too.

Inform them that professionals who work to help rehabilitate persons with brain injury are aware that rehabilitation is a unique experience for them and their families. They may be surprised to learn that most people receiving rehabilitation have sentiments similar to those expressed above. To prepare them for the emotions that they may experience during rehabilitation, it is important to understand what rehabilitation is – and is not – and what it can – and cannot – accomplish. Let them know that by better understanding rehabilitation they will find that they can have more say in how their care proceeds.

Teaching the Nature of Rehabilitation

You can boil down a lot of concern about rehabilitation for persons with brain injury by using two insights. Rehabilitation differs from most other health care in two fundamental ways:

- The goal of rehabilitation is to facilitate their function and teach them how to compensate, not to cure injury or illness.

- Rehabilitation requires their participation.

These two simple statements are at the heart of all rehabilitation. Yet, if they fail to appreciate their implications, they will be frustrated with the care they get.

Begin by exploring the meaning for them of the first statement. Most health care strives to accomplish different goals in treatment than does rehabilitation. Summarize for them that much of traditional health care has as its goal to cure or fix a problem using these examples:

- Physicians set broken legs to fix the break.

- Wounds are cleaned and sutured so that they heal.

- Medications cure infections.

In contrast, most of the symptoms for which people come to rehabilitation are not curable: brain injury is a classic example. Professionals are unable to "fix," or cure, brain injury. Hence, the goal of rehabilitation is to facilitate brain function so that their deficits are reduced or so that they learn to use other parts of their brain to compensate (i.e., accomplish the same task in a different manner) for the injured part. Highlighting this difference for them is crucial.

Suggest that rehabilitation may be the first phase of treatment after their injury in which their health care providers discuss recovery in terms of deficit reduction and compensation rather than curing them. This may be as shocking to them as it is to most people. The contrast in this regard between acute treatment and rehabilitation treatment can be overwhelming.

It may be the first time they realize that their recovery may be incomplete. Inquire if they and their family may even have been told at the initial acute hospital that they were "going to be fine." Many people with brain injury and their families breathe a sigh of relief upon being told "you are going to be fine," taking the words literally to mean "complete recovery." Now in rehabilitation they may be realizing that the message is different.

To address any confusion, they should be clear about their expectations. Refer to the exercise in the companion book. Have them complete the exercise to see what their expectations were coming to rehabilitation.

So as to decrease any resentment at previous caregivers whose message about recovery is no longer being trumpeted by rehabilitation professionals, it is important to help them understand acute professionals. Those professionals are often involved in saving lives and they do miraculous work. However, many acute-care professionals:

- Are trained to fix and cure problems.

- Usually give out good news.

- May be emotionally unprepared themselves to tell them news that might distress persons with brain injury.

- Mean they will likely be able to "walk and talk," though without specifying how well, when they say "You are going to be all right."

- Do not follow people for years to know how their predictions play out and they may believe the persons with brain injury will be fine.

Empathize with the persons with brain injury that when their rehabilitation team begins to discuss limitations it can be very disappointing. Many people even complain that they have been told that everything will be okay. They may experience considerable disbelief or even anger when their rehabilitation team disagrees with the messages they have been given in acute care.

Assure them that their team will work to minimize their eventual limitations, sometimes called residual deficits, and maximize their abilities, but some problems may be permanent. They should make sure their team knows about their feelings and reactions to messages the team is giving them, so they can work together more effectively.

Refer to the exercise in the companion book. To help accomplish this have them complete the exercise and suggest that they share it with their rehabilitation therapists.

Despite being told that their recovery may not be complete, make sure that they do *not* take this to mean that they should abandon hope. Emphasize that their attitude and effort can greatly affect their eventual abilities. This should bring you to a discussion of the second difference between traditional care and rehabilitation: their effort is crucial.

Before proceeding to address this, show them the following box and have them refer to it throughout this Lesson.

YOUR EFFORT MAKES A HUGE

DIFFERENCE IN YOUR OUTCOME!

Highlight that their effort makes a huge difference in their outcome. Explain that in other aspects of health care this is less true using two examples:

- When they take medications, so long as they take the medications as prescribed, the chemistry of the pill requires little from them.

- When they have surgery, they passively lie on the surgical table.

However, in rehabilitation they must work to get results. Their therapists will require them to do physical structured activities to improve their strength, coordination, balance, sensation, etc. Therapists will need them to do guided mental tasks to enhance thinking, reasoning, concentration, memory, and awareness.

Instruct the persons with brain injury that the job of therapists is to:

- Design retraining and compensation techniques for them.

- Provide them with the right exercises — physical and mental — to retrain them or teach them to compensate.

- Guide them in doing the exercises.

- Give them "homework" to practice between treatment sessions.

Note for them that the therapists are not doing things *to* them in the manner that medications or surgery do.

Prepare them to understand that rehabilitation therapists may push them to thoroughly participate during rehabilitation because the results depend on their efforts. Contrast for them that a physical therapist in an Intensive Care Unit may move their leg to help maintain its movement, but a physical therapist in rehabilitation is more likely to teach them exercises to perform to strengthen their leg.

Utilize Box 3.1 in the companion book to show the differences between traditional care and rehabilitation.

Guide them that there is a *potential* for limitations and that they must actively engage in rehabilitation to reduce them. Encourage them to stay positive and focused on doing the best they can in rehabilitation to improve their results. In fact, it is valuable to have them write down their new goals, other than being cured, for rehabilitation in terms of improvement and limiting residual problems.

To accomplish this, have them complete the exercise in the book for persons with brain injury.

Tell them that the best advice from experienced rehabilitation professionals is to maintain hope, work as hard as they can to achieve their vision of recovery and fulfill that hope, while planning to make necessary life changes, if they must. It is unwise to have them put all of their eggs in one basket: instead, believe – have faith and avoid giving up, on one hand; but be realistic – plan for various outcomes, on the other hand.

Facilitating Acceptance of Emotional Help During Rehabilitation

Acknowledge for them that the preceding section may have been very difficult. They may have found that it challenged their previous concept of their expected care. They are normal if they find that confronting their existing concepts was distressing.

Make sure they know that they are not alone. Centers that specialize in rehabilitation typically include psychologists as part of their treatment team. In fact, it is often routine that *everyone* sees a psychologist because the process of rehabilitation is so challenging.

Prepare them that seeing a psychologist is recognition of how emotionally challenging it can be to have a brain injury, but it does not imply that they are weak or mentally ill. Rather, grief is normal, but people tend to handle significant life changes better when they can discuss them with others.

Suggest that their psychologist can act as an expert source of information and can give them perspectives garnered from having listened to other people with brain injury. You can compare this to explorers going into the unknown using scouts who had been there before; their psychologist is their emotional scout, having learned which ideas work for persons with brain injury and which ones increase distress: their psychologist knows the emotional landscape of brain injury, just like a scout knows physical geography. Encourage them to use their psychologist to emotionally prepare themselves for their journey into the unknown turf of rehabilitation and brain injury.

Let them know that their psychologist may come to visit them early during their rehabilitation:

- This is to establish rapport and to learn about them.

- This provides a head start on helping them cope in the future, if they find that rehabilitation and brain injury are overwhelming.

- It helps the psychologist know them so that the psychologist can assist their family members who may need support themselves.

Also, they may be offered follow-up visits after discharge since the process of grieving often extends beyond rehabilitation. Of course, they and their psychologist may decide that they are coping adequately with little professional support and minimum help is necessary. Advise them that it still is wise to maintain contact should this change in the future.

Let them know that in addition to the rehabilitation team psychologist, there are other providers who can help them with emotional coping. They may find that they emotionally connect with lots of team members: physicians, nurses, therapists, chaplains, social workers, etc. Tell them to avail themselves of the guidance and knowledge of their whole team and blend perspectives to fit their needs.

To ready them for discussion with their psychologist, it may be helpful to have them write down concerns they want to discuss with their psychologist so that they do not forget them. Refer them to the form in Box 3.2.

Assisting Clients in Getting Comfortable in Rehabilitation

Persons with brain injury may find that it is difficult to stay positive when they first arrive on the rehabilitation unit. They are in an unfamiliar environment with people they do not know. It is common for people to feel uncertain and worried.

Discuss with them that in such circumstances they may seek to apply their own familiar routines only to find that the rehabilitation center has its own procedures. Assure them that it is all right to discuss with their providers how they like things done so as to feel most comfortable. Many rehabilitation processes are flexible and their team should strive to meet their desires. Make sure they know, however, that some procedures are set to accommodate everyone in the rehabilitation program or to maximize their recovery, and there may be less flexibility for those procedures.

To help them sort these out, have them complete the exercise in the companion book.

If they are unhappy about the rehabilitation routine, instruct them to talk with their team (i.e., nurses, therapists, psychologist, social worker, physician). They can show the staff the proceeding exercise and their answers to facilitate understanding. Also, have them ask for certain written materials that can help give them more control.[1] Tell them to ask for a:

- Schedule of therapies and unit activities

- List of their team members, their jobs, and their phone numbers (they may also want to ask for team members' business cards)

- Memory notebook or day planner to record their activities so that they can recall what they have been doing in treatment and can establish a sense of continuity which will make them feel more in control

- Copy of visiting hours

- Visitors' log book so that family and other visitors can write entries and persons with brain injury can review the visits after people leave, to extend the emotional support

- Calendar for their room

- Hospital map

---

[1] Note that they are also entitled to various items by law, such as a Patient Bill of Rights, which are typically posted on their rehabilitation unit. If they want a copy, have them ask their social worker for a copy of any legally mandated material.

Have them use the form in Box 3.3 in the companion book, to remember to ask for the items listed above, and have them complete the form in Box 3.4, to write down their team members.

Let the persons with brain injury know that many of the concerns covered in this Lesson can be addressed during family conferences. Rehabilitation centers usually will schedule periodic meetings with them, their family, and their team to make sure that the professionals attend to any issues they and their family may have. The team will also tell them concerns the team has.

However, advise them to not wait to voice their worries, or their hopes, to their team. Instruct them that, in fact, their team may hold staff-only meetings more frequently than family conferences. Have the persons with brain injury plan to ask when the staff meetings or rounds are held. It is often useful to pose questions to their team before those meetings so that all of their team members can confer on how to meet their needs.

Coping with Wanting to Leave the Rehabilitation Center

As rehabilitation proceeds, insecurity may still remain. They may be worried about how they are doing or how far they will progress. Tell them to ask their team since insecurity increases in an information vacuum. As they proceed through rehabilitation, hopefully their sense of security will increase. Remind them that their therapists, nurses, etc., will become familiar.

Yet, one large doubt may remain: "When will I be discharged?" This question can have two opposite meanings:

- "How soon can I go home?"
- "They can't discharge me; I'm not ready to go home!"

If they experience either of these sentiments, they are having natural reactions to rehabilitation. Inquire of them which sentiment underlies this question. If it is the former, introduce the topic of treatment purposes, processes, and goals, particularly cognitive therapy.

Understanding Cognitive Treatment

They may feel that rehabilitation treatment, particularly the cognitive therapies to improve memory and reasoning, seem silly; the exercises look childish. This can stem from the fact that on the surface the tasks appear like childhood games or activities.

Explain that typically the therapists are trying to stimulate certain parts of the brain. Some of these simple appearing tasks do that because they require use of specific brain areas, whereas complex tasks utilize broad areas of the brain. Let them know that it all right to ask their therapists about the purposes of any cognitive exercise. (You can help by relating that in the real world they use their whole brain, but if therapists only gave them real-world activities to do, there would be less attention paid to areas of difficulty.) Actually, a combination of specific brain tasks and application to real-world activities is most common.

Still, even many of the real-world activities that therapists focus on may seem like they would be below their level of functioning before their injury. Empathize that it is hard to work on things that they knew how to do before and that they thought they were done learning to do: they learned them in the past when they were younger and it can be frustrating to cover the same ground again.

Discuss with them that best practices in rehabilitation have therapists requiring them to show that they can do things now, not just that they could do them before their injury. Otherwise, therapists might assume they actually have skills that may have been affected by their injury and they will leave rehabilitation without the abilities they need. It is difficult to spend time in their life relearning things, particularly thinking skills, but it is wise to take advantage of the time in rehabilitation to get as much back as they can.

Responsibilities at Home

Another reason for possible frustration with hospitalization is that there are real-world responsibilities they feel driven to get back to handling: paying bills, returning to work, repairing things in their house, etc. If this underlies their desire to leave, they may be annoyed with their rehabilitation team because the team seems to attend insufficiently to their concerns about those things. You can suggest that the likely reason for the therapists' focus on treatment rather than their life before their injury is that the therapists believe their brain is not yet capable of handling these responsibilities *well*.

Ask the persons with brain injury to consider that their therapists may be protecting them from prematurely attempting tasks that will go poorly based on data about them specifically and their teams' experience working with people who came before them, in general. While it can make them very angry, it is wise for them to remember that their team's insistence that they continue in rehabilitation reflects a desire for them to do well *after* discharge.

Let them know that to protect them sometimes therapists will:

- Prohibit an activity (e.g., driving)
- Insist on their being supervised after discharge
- Advise them to delay return to work (so they do not get fired because they returned too soon before their full skills were back)
- Stay in the rehabilitation center so that they *succeed* when they do return to the real world

Such restrictions should be conceptualized for persons with brain injury as steps to buy them time to recover and be safe.

Another idea to suggest is for them to think of it as a positive sign when their team wants them to continue in treatment because it means that their therapists believe they can benefit and get better. A couple of more weeks in rehabilitation may mean a much easier time for the rest of their life; after all, when they are 90 years old looking back on their life they probably will not regret having worked a few weeks less now because they were in rehabilitation, but they may regret not having taken advantage of treatment that was available to them that could have made their life better.

Trusting Expert Advice

Finally, irritability with having to stay in the rehabilitation center may reflect their misperceiving the extent of their injury. You should make certain that you know how they perceive their injury: mild, severe, nonexistent, etc. Ask them what strengths and deficits they perceive themselves to have. There may be a difference between their self-perception and the view of other people.

If they downplay their difficulties, do not be surprised. It is difficult to see one's own memory, judgment, or reasoning problems. Their brain may appear fine to them. For example, it may tell them that they are recalling everything because it fails to realize how much it forgot!

However, their therapists and family may see the problem. Trusting their rehabilitation team in such circumstances is crucial, but it is difficult to trust these professionals whom they have only known briefly. Perhaps the best way to consider this situation is to have them think of their team as experts who they have hired to advise them about cognition (i.e., thinking, reasoning, memory) and the implications of problems in these areas.

Remind them that they trust experts they barely know – if at all – all of the time: an airline pilot, the people who built the bridge they drive over, the elevator manufacturer, etc. It seems harder in rehabilitation because their own cognition seems like something they should be the expert about – in contrast, they know they can't fly an airplane – so they have less faith when the rehabilitation team gives them information that is contrary to what their own brain tells them. Still, suggest that the next time they look at a big jet liner think about this: Does their brain *really* tell them that great big metal thing will *fly*?

The Flip Side: Worried About Leaving Rehabilitation

Eventually their team will tell them it is time to leave. They may feel panic. Surprisingly, the rehabilitation center may have become a source of comfort. Everyone accepts them. They see other people addressing difficulties similar to theirs. Everything is physically accessible (e.g., doorways, bathrooms, counter heights). There are nurses to help with activities of daily living. However, the real world can be a scary place. If they are fearful, step in to provide reassurance.

You can again frame this as an issue of trust. Their caregivers want them to succeed. Encourage them to tell their therapists if they feel that they will have needs after discharge that have been inadequately addressed. If they are afraid, tell them to tell the therapists that, too. Acknowledge the range of emotions that they experience as they pass through rehabilitation and face leaving.

Make sure they know to discuss their worries early with their team, rather than waiting until the last minute. If they know their concerns, therapists will often arrange for practice experiences for the things they are concerned about (e.g., outings with therapists outside of the hospital or therapeutic passes to go home with family). Make sure they or their family keep a log to return to the therapists of successful activities they attempt during passes, and the hurdles they encounter while on passes that need addressing. They can use the form in Box 3.5 to record these.

Remind them, too, that once they go home the rehabilitation center does not vanish. They can always come for an appointment to get advice. In truth, it is best to advise them to schedule some automatic follow-up visits with their rehabilitation physician, psychologist, and therapists before discharge. Typically at discharge, they will receive discharge instructions that include follow-up visits and appointments for ongoing therapy. They can use the form in Box 3.6 to record their follow-up visits.

Advising Persons with Brain Injury About Their Family and Their Rehabilitation

Families Who Are Involved

Family members may experience unique challenges during the rehabilitation period. It is important that persons with brain injury realize the role their family can play in their rehabilitation and be comfortable with their involvement.

One factor that confuses family members is that rehabilitation rarely proceeds without starts and stops. Ideally, every day would be better than the preceding one. In reality, persons with brain injury may have setbacks. On any given day they may appear as they had a few days, or even weeks, earlier. Factors such as a poor night's sleep, a stressful day, poor appetite, etc., may affect them more than they might expect or more than such things would have influenced them before their injury. Brain injury can change their sensitivity to these influences.

You can direct persons with brain injury to realize that family members are trying to discern progress and that days in which they do poorly can be traumatic. Since their family members are often keenly aware of fluctuations in abilities, you can encourage them to tell their families to seek reassurance from the treatment team so that family members can understand which fluctuations they should accept as part of natural variations during rehabilitation and which symptoms ought to be of concern. If the family understands the natural process of rehabilitation, they may apply less pressure to persons with brain injury during an off day—so long as it is just a day—once in awhile.

Point out that feeling comfortable with their family talking with their team is valuable because families may detect changes worth noting for the team. Their family knew them before their injury and they may be closely monitoring their status, so they may detect changes before the team. Consultation between their family and their team can help both do the best job for them.

Families Who Are Struggling to Understand

Their family, however, may struggle to accurately perceive their capabilities. This is true even when persons with brain injury are putting forth their best effort. For example, if persons with brain injury have trouble with initiation (e.g., starting activities, realizing they should do something, making plans) their family may sometimes believe they are lazy. Note for the persons with brain injury that this typically reflects that their family is trying to understand their behavior as if they did not have a brain injury. Of course, they can be lazy *and* have a brain injury, but other reasons may apply for their behavior due to their brain injury.

Note for them that their family is probably unfamiliar with reasons for their behavior that are rooted in brain injury and their family may express disappointment with them. In such instances you can help the persons with brain injury be less frustrated with their family.

Inquire whether persons with brain injury are feeling distress, guilt, or shame based on family reactions. Open discussion about the reasons for these feelings, including disclosures about their effort, their expectations, and their history before injury, can help avoid hurt feelings. If they believe their family is struggling to understand how hard it is for them to put forth their best effort, then you could suggest they talk with their team about their family's perception.

Similar problems can arise in regard to cognitive functioning. Their family may relate that their deficits are typical for them – "He always had a poor memory" or "She was never good at drawing" or "Math was never his strong suit." Any of these statements may, in part, be true. Nevertheless, when therapists determine that there are cognitive difficulties, therapists do so by using extensive data bases to judge performance and are looking at variations greater than those found in people without injuries—beyond what would be normal variations of being good or bad at something prior to having an injury.

Their family may report that they see no change from before their injury, despite reports by therapists to the contrary. This is difficult for persons with brain injury to handle since they become torn between family and therapist input. Differences in viewpoint arise most commonly in regard to memory functioning. Explain to persons with brain injury that:

- The discrepancy often occurs because of the complexity of memory functioning. Brain injury usually affects memory for new information, whereas memory for more distant events is sometimes spared. When therapists assess new learning, they detect deficits, but when their family discusses events in their life from before the injury, they seem fine.

- Families sometimes word questions to them that imply the correct answer and they provide enough information in the question so that persons with brain injury can answer.

- Sometimes persons with brain injury answer questions with a "yes" or "no," appearing to be accurately recalling, whereas they are just responding to the information cue families gave them.

- Family members may accept a partial answer, filling in the missing information, assuming they really knew the full answer. They assume persons with brain injury knew more than they said!

All of this can lead to great misunderstandings. Frustration between them, their family, and their team can begin because everyone has a different perception of their abilities. It would seem, therefore, that the best advice you can give them to help cope with differing opinions is to quickly recognize when they and their family disagree about their functioning or when there is a difference with their team. Then, recommend that information should be exchanged between their family and their team so that all agree and are working from the same foundation.

Summary

Brain injury is an emotional experience. It can induce fear, worry, depression, anxiety, hopelessness, disbelief, mistrust, frustration, anger, guilt, despair, and grief. Rehabilitation can, at its worse, increase these feelings, or, at its best, lessen them. Rehabilitation can be a period of reassurance, hope, belief, trust, growth, renewal, and faith. You can facilitate the positive nature of rehabilitation by helping persons with brain injury address the process of rehabilitation and some of its challenges. It is normal for persons with brain injury to grieve during (and after) rehabilitation; it is natural for them to experience a sense of loss and it is typical to see new possibilities in their future. Provide support when persons with brain injury experience a range of emotions, all of which are normal, and advance information for wise decision making to enhance rehabilitation.

Lesson 4   *Emotional Responses to Brain Injury—Reclaiming Grief*

Overview

The overarching goal of Lesson 4 is to introduce clients with brain injury to the range of emotional responses that are possible following this injury. Normalizing the multitude of possible feelings of variable intensity may help reduce fear about changes that clients with brain injury struggle to deal with and accept. In Lesson 4, the real stories featured in Lesson 1 are used to supplement and guide applications and exercises. In addition, up-to-date information from the scientific psychiatric and brain-injury literatures is incorporated into the Lesson content. Therapists should assist clients in identifying, accepting, and managing their own feelings and concerns related to their brain injury and associated losses.

Rationale

1. Persons with brain injury experience rapidly fluctuating, intense emotions and other feelings. Providing them with an anchor and telling them that these are expected reactions and phenomena after brain injury can be reassuring and prevent a catastrophic reaction.

2. Normalizing grief feelings but explaining how to tell if they need to seek medical help for a possible depression will help clients self-monitor and take care of themselves during adjustment.

Presenting the Goals of This Lesson

Using the stories from Lesson 1 that describe experiences of real individuals with brain injury and their families, explain to clients that you will focus more this time on the feelings, struggles, and losses that each of them experienced. Indicate that you will show them how these emotional responses are common markers during the journey of persons who have brain injury.

Review the following goals for this Lesson with clients.

- Identify and accept your own feelings and worries related to your brain injury experience and recovery

- Improve self-management of feelings and worries related to your brain injury

- Adopt a positive view of your post-injury emotions and concerns

- Understand the complexity of coping with brain injury

Loss Is a Part of Having a Brain Injury

Lesson 4 describes both typical and pathological emotional responses to the losses related to brain injury and attempts to instill hope for a positive, productive outcome. Explain that loss is a part of the brain injury experience and that you will be using stories from Lesson 1 to illustrate this idea for clients. Before beginning to review the stories, tell clients that the comments in Box 4.1, Lesson 4 of their books are from individuals with brain injury and their families and are often heard on the typical inpatient or outpatient brain injury rehabilitation unit. Direct clients to look at both Box 1.1 of Lesson 1, and Box 4.1 of Lesson 4, which are the same. Take time to emphasize that the feelings, struggles, and losses that are quoted in the Box are said often by people and their family members who are beginning the life-long journey of recovering and living with brain injury.

Call clients' attention to the boldfaced words in Box 4.1 to help emphasize these commonly reported losses and feelings following brain injury.

Tell them that, as they work through Lesson 4, they will learn that while persons with brain injury are three times more likely to develop depression than persons without injury, normal grief over losses from the brain injury can also explain sadness during recovery. Tell them that Lesson 4 will provide them with information about how to know whether the emotional and behavioral reactions they are having are normal or whether they should seek help in coping to make progress in their recovery more likely.

Begin review of the stories from Lesson 1 with clients, emphasizing the italicized, bolded words that represent emotional reactions and thoughts each of the main characters are having.

Revisiting Brian's Story

Brian was driving home from an out-of-state business trip late one evening. The next thing he knew he was in a hospital bed with a headache. The strangers around him identified themselves as nurses or therapists. He had been in a serious motor vehicle accident and was in brain injury rehabilitation, he was told. He ***struggled to fight crushing fatigue*** to organize his thoughts, think, and remember even a little of what had happened to him. He asked person after person, "Where am I?" "What happened to me?" When staff or relatives told him what happened, he found that he soon forgot what they had told him and had to ask again. He ***became irritated*** with those around him because they were having trouble understanding what he was saying for some reason. His family and the medical staff told him that a passing motorist had reported seeing his car in a gully. His car appeared to police to have drifted off the highway. He learned that his head struck the dashboard, resulting in a subarachnoid hemorrhage in the left side of his brain. Brian was determined to remember the cause of his accident. He asked everyone for clues but no one knew. He got a nurse to find a version of the police report in his medical chart admission papers. It was agonizingly short on details. "Male, 40's, status post single car crash, found with LOC (loss of consciousness) slumped forward on dash of his vehicle, 2:45 a.m. Left forehead laceration. Male transported to trauma center via medical rescue helicopter." As his thinking began to clear, Brian became aware of a weakness in his right hand and leg. *He was annoyed* as nurses and therapists told him not to get up without help, not to go to the bathroom without first calling them, that he couldn't have a drink of water until his swallowing test, and that he had to stay out of bed. When he tried to get up anyway, he was wobbly and had to grab furniture to avoid falling. One time he fell. Finding it hard to hide the *frustration in their voices,* staff were constantly telling him not to get up or yelling, "Sit down!" At times Brian found himself wearing a cotton jacket that was tied to a chair so he couldn't get up. Staff would occasionally use soft arm bands to keep him restrained in his bed or chair, saying "it is to keep you safe." As he tried to ask questions or express his feelings and thoughts he noticed that it was very *hard to get his words to come out clearly*. Brian's wife and son treated him as if he were being rude or acting like a child. Though he could not figure out why, *they seemed overwhelmed, confused, embarrassed, and frustrated by him*. All Brian wanted to do was sleep, have people leave him alone, and find out what happened to him and why *he didn't feel like himself anymore.*

Symptoms and Trials

Tell clients that Brian's experience is quite common after a brain injury. Persons with brain injury often report they feel at first like they are in a fog. Fatigue is frequently a constant companion. Speech may be confused, slurred, and faint. It may be hard to understand the speech of others. The brain injury can cause a range of typical impairments in thinking skills, especially memory and reasoning. Persons with brain injury thus *struggle to make sense out of their situation*. They may *feel restless, on an emotional roller coaster, and not as able to tolerate even minor frustrations.* They can snap at those close to them. They may be unsafe because they do not realize their limitations. *Fear of loss of independence and control* can drive them to rebel against staff and family who are trying to keep them safe.

Fortunately, before the end of our story, help becomes available in several forms for both Brian and his family. We continue Brian's story to show a typical recovery path. Brian's story, and this book, will also make clear how persons with brain injury and their family members can find and access healing and helpful resources. Many people, for example, receive both inpatient and outpatient rehabilitation services following their brain injury.

Hope and Healing

Brian's initial inpatient rehabilitation was provided by a team of specialists including a physician, social worker, neuropsychologist, physical therapist, speech language pathologist, occupational therapist, recreational therapist, and nurse specialist. He was ***given medication temporarily*** to help him sleep better at night and stay awake and alert during the day therapies. He made excellent progress with his walking and was able to leave the hospital with only a cane for assistance for balance. His rehabilitation program included physical therapies as well as education. He spent at least one, and sometimes two sessions a day with the neuropsychologist, social worker, occupational therapist, and speech therapist learning about his injury as well as practicing memory and thinking strategies. The team of therapists also trained him to monitor and control his behavior consistently so he could be less impulsive, safe, and appropriate with others. ***Counseling was helping him, and his family, understand and accept the challenges*** resulting from his brain injury. His characteristic kind and caring ways were slowly returning to his daily interactions with family and friends.

Brian was fortunate to also receive outpatient rehabilitation. Many people, like Brian, transfer from inpatient to outpatient rehabilitation in a fairly short period of time—two weeks to one month. Like Brian, they make progress in inpatient brain injury rehabilitation, but may still have some problems to work on. Outpatient therapy teams usually do a new assessment or evaluation of the person with the brain injury. They often have a report from the inpatient team. So the outpatient therapists compare their new evaluation findings with the old report to get an accurate picture of clients' current skills and abilities. The outpatient team then sets new goals based on the new evaluation because these new goals can then reflect the next step in recovery. Over the next 12 months, a typical time frame for most persons following discharge from an inpatient brain injury unit, Brian's outpatient rehabilitation therapists began to get him ready to resume work. He was able to obtain a job through his state's department of rehabilitation services. A job "coach" went to work with him for a while to help problem solve any barriers to Brian's becoming a productive worker. With *family support*, and *gentle guidance from helpers to become more self-aware*, Brian has managed *to regain much of what he lost* and is successfully relying on new ideas for coping.

Learning from Brian's Story

Ask clients to explain what Brian's story says to them about emotional responses following brain injury and coping effectively. Show clients that Brian was *annoyed, frustrated, and afraid*. He had to work very hard not to give in to being *tired*. Point out that his family was having normal feelings related to the changes in their lives because of Brian's brain injury and how it made him different from the person they knew. Brian chose to really work hard in rehabilitation, taking advantage of every opportunity to get training and help. Make the point for clients that Brian's strategy, and his positive outlook, his coping choice of sticking with rehabilitation and work in spite of his being tired and frustrated, and his wonderful family support really paid off. He was able to work again and have a satisfying life situation, even though he still has ups and downs.

Looking Back at Pat's Story

Review the story below with clients, pointing out the bolded, italicized words and phrases.

After seven months, Pat finally made an appointment to take her three children to see a therapist. She needed help with parenting. Since her car accident almost one year ago, family life had become chaotic. Everyday chores seemed *overwhelming* to Pat. Her ability to manage had been dwindling and she was *losing her temper* more and more frequently with the kids. She couldn't get the 6-year-old to sleep in her own bed. The 10- and 13-year-olds were fighting with each other and baiting the youngest until she cried. They all refused to do what she asked them to do. Her husband was also recovering from neck, back, and leg injuries, so could not manage them well either.

Pat's return to work, eight months after the accident, brought the behavioral and parenting challenges at home to a crisis point. With the advice of a friend Pat made an appointment with a local family therapist. The psychologist took one look at the waiting room full of out-of-control children, the **passive and bewildered** mother, and asked Pat to come in first. During the interview, the psychologist began to ask a lot of questions about the accident. Pat reported what doctors, nurses, and family members told her, explaining to the psychologist that she herself could not really recall a thing. She and her husband were coming home from a wonderful New Year's Eve dinner at a local restaurant when their car was hit broadside by a pizza delivery truck. As a result of the impact, her husband's right shoulder pushed into her left chest, breaking eight of her ribs and collapsing a lung. Both of them were feared near death. They had to be cut out of their car and were rushed to a local hospital trauma center.

Doctors in the emergency room quickly sent Pat up to the Operating Room where surgeons worked to re-inflate her lung and remove her spleen. The final physician's summary stated that most of the couples' injuries were in their chest and extremities and that they would eventually recover. Family members took care of the children for the three weeks that she and her husband were in the hospital and for the two months they were ambulating with crutches at home. Pat and her husband were *in pain* and on various pain medications for a long time. The *youngest child was tearful, anxious, and clingy*. She refused to sleep in her own bed.

Pat was very happy to return to work. However, Pat, once known for her organization and time management in running a busy household of five and holding down a demanding managerial job, **did not seem to have any energy** or skills anymore. Details began to slip through her fingers. Major mistakes became frequent, both at the office and at home. Dinner did not seem to get on the table regularly. The children were not getting to bed on time. All her husband wanted to do was take his pain medication and sleep. He had applied for and received disability insurance and was not able to return to work.

After talking with Pat and administering some cognitive tests, the psychologist finally met with all of them. She referred Pat to a neurologist, reporting to Pat that the test results suggested that the accident may have caused a brain injury, perhaps not known at the time. Pat and her children were told about brain injury symptoms and given printed information from the Brain Injury Association of America (www.biausa.org). As it turned out, Pat was later diagnosed with a moderately severe anoxic brain injury caused by a lack of oxygen to her brain at the time of the accident. She was referred for and went through outpatient rehabilitation. She learned strategies for coping with her memory problems and was able to resume her job on a part-time basis. She improved her parenting skills, though she required parenting help with and counseling for her children. Fortunately her family had the financial resources to provide the help she needed.

Learning from Pat's Story

Ask clients what can be learned about losses, emotions, and successful coping after brain injury from Pat's story. Point out for clients that Pat had to wait a long time to get reassurance about what she was feeling and experiencing because doctors did not notice her brain injury right away. She and her family members were overwhelmed, worried, and confused about her daily mistakes and coping problems. Point out for clients that Pat had anger and frustration. She did not understand what was wrong with her and took out her frustration on her children. The children reacted with misbehavior and anxiety. Make the take-home points of this story clear for clients by summarizing that Pat's trust of her instincts and her quest for help made all the difference for her recovery. She was referred to a professional who knew about brain injury symptoms and challenges. The professional gave Pat and her family the information and recommendations they needed. Finally, Pat started on the right path to recovery. She and her family were able to work back toward a better life together, despite Pat's brain injury. Conclude for clients that information, professional support and guidance, and use of helpful coping can lead to improvements and progress even if a person gets a delayed start in dealing with a brain injury. Pat's love of her family, trust in her instincts, and her discovery of a professional skilled and knowledgeable in helping persons with brain injury were the primary factors in dealing with her losses and emotions in a successful manner.

Revisiting Audrey and John's Story

Review the story with clients, again pointing out the bolded, italicized words and phrases and making relevant comments to underscore the primary concepts for clients to remember.

At 5 p.m. Audrey knew her husband was nearing home after one of his truck runs up the coast. Tonight she did not receive his usual CB-radio call telling her he was almost there. Instead a highway patrolman arrived to tell her John had been taken to a hospital about one hour away. She threw on her coat, called her mother to come watch their 6-year-old twins, and took off for the emergency room.

Audrey heard from the emergency room staff that a passing motorist notified police that John was driving slowly and weaving all over the road. John actually was able to radio his company dispatcher to tell her he was feeling sick, pull his truck over, and put on the brake, before collapsing on the steering wheel. Hospital staff worked to stabilize John. A scan revealed an aneurysm, a small "bubble" of one of the blood vessels in his brain, had burst. A team of surgeons operated to drain the blood, removing a piece of his skull to prevent further damage from swelling. Audrey was ***overjoyed to see her husband*** when they finally took John back to his room in Neuroscience Intensive Care. The helmet covering the exposed portion of his head was a constant reminder of how close a call this was.

John was quiet for a few days, receiving nutrition and medicine from tubes and IVs. Then he started to move restlessly. He would open his eyes when Audrey called his name but close them again quickly. ***"Does he still know me?" Audrey wondered***. John's days and nights were mixed up. He was up at night and wanted to sleep during the day. The few words he spoke were scrambled or mixed up. Despite being told to leave his helmet on, he kept trying to take it off. He pulled out his IV twice. Audrey ***missed her twins*** but tried to stay with John at night while her mother was at home with the children. ***She was exhausted*** *during the day*, trying to keep up with her sons. ***John was embarrassing her***. He tried to grab the nurses and ask them for kisses. He was demanding and ungrateful toward Audrey. He pleaded for her to take him home and became ***enraged*** when she said she could not.

John's progress was slow, and he was moved to a nursing home for a time. His behavior improved, but he still acted like a child much of the time. Audrey was able to be home with her children more, but she missed her partner and spouse. Finances nearing collapse, Audrey took a part-time job. She was forced to learn about the banking and finances, and ***struggled to find out what she could*** about community resources for her husband's return. ***She fought her own depression***, especially when friends and relatives told her "You should be grateful he survived!" It was difficult for her to be the loving, helpful wife when this man she married now seemed like a stranger.

Learning from John and Audrey's Story

Ask clients what they can learn about losses, emotions, and successful coping after brain injury from John and Audrey's story. Point out that John was not very aware of his behavior for some time, and as is often the case, his family had difficulty coping with his injury-related changes. As time went on medication, counseling, rehabilitation therapies, and hard work made the difference. Tell clients that John and Audrey's story shows that having patience, acceptance, and counting any blessings that are available are critical for making progress in recovery and readjustment after a brain injury.

Tell clients that you are now going to look more closely at the range of normal emotional responses to brain injury. Direct them to Box 4.2 of Lesson 4 in their books and help them read about the many feelings experienced after brain injury by both the person who has the brain injury and their family members.

Strive to give clients a clear picture of the complexity of coping after brain injury. Using Box 4.2, discuss the concept that brain injury-related losses are so hard to deal with because of thinking, memory, language, and coping impairments that result from the injury. Go on to explain that persons recovering from any injury or disability can encounter coping hurdles. However, brain injury is different from other disabilities because the coping has to occur using a brain that is injured while for other injuries, such as to the spinal cord, the coping is usually undertaken with an intact brain.

Point out for clients that as one consequence, among many, of trying to cope using their injured brain, persons with the brain injury may alienate or communicate ineffectively with the very supporters that are crucial for their eventual recovery and successful return to the community. Point out that Lesson 2 provided some specific compensatory strategies for communication and other common cognitive deficits following brain injury to help bolster coping resources and make it more likely that the injured brain will cope effectively. Therapists should help clients with brain injury understand and normalize their common postinjury emotions. Explain that for persons with brain injury, whether they have lost the use of their arms, memory, legs, speech, or vision, the injury is bound to have a great impact on their life and feelings. Note that the last thing they may remember before the accident or illness was being at work, school, or at home. Later, perhaps after being in a coma for weeks, they probably found themselves in a hospital. Tell clients that in a minute, people can often go from being totally independent to needing someone else to help them take care of even their most basic bodily functions. In the early days of recovery, and even later, persons with brain injury may be in tremendous pain. Mention to clients that they may be wondering why they no longer feel like themselves, and may not know who that "self" is now. Feelings and emotions may flow with worrisome speed and unpredictability. Tell clients that they may find it frightening when family members and others closest to them appear confused about how to help them figure things out. Reassure clients about the good news that all of these feelings and experiences are common and reported by almost all people who have experienced a brain injury.

If there is a family member, partner, or friend of the person with the brain injury present, direct clients' attention to the specific material about family members in Box 4.2, explaining that many persons close to those who have sustained a brain injury face their own significant changes and challenges in the wake of the injury. Tell clients that you will review several examples of common difficulties that family members experience. In addition, mention that Lesson 7 will provide more detailed information about the challenges and feelings of family members and caregivers of persons with brain injury. Tell clients that family members frequently describe their own emotional roller coaster. Relief and gratitude for the survival of their loved one can quickly become sadness, fear, or even anger when they notice some unpleasant changes in the personality and behavior of the person they nearly lost. Family members may also have to face the reality that the role of the primary wage earner in the family may be too difficult to resume. A spouse or partner who never handled the family finances may now have to scramble to learn in order to avoid financial ruin following rising medical expenses and no income. Mention that marriages and families can be unbalanced and disrupted when the persons with brain injury lose the capacity to take care of themselves and to make decisions. Adult children from a prior marriage, for example, may enter the picture and try to take the primary role in managing their parent's situation, disrupting the relationship with the parent's new spouse. Finally, therapists should explain that family members and friends report feeling loss of intimacy when nurses must now provide most of the physical care for their spouse or partner.

Good News

The therapist should reassure clients that there are several pieces of good news in this Lesson, and the entire book. First, this Lesson and those that follow will show them that most of the emotions they are having are grief-related and normal for individuals and their family members who have losses associated with brain injury. That is not to say that recovery and coping are easy. In particular, Lesson 4 will tell them how to know when their symptoms and behaviors are becoming disruptive and self-defeating to the point that they should seek help. Second, the Lessons will guide them toward coping adaptively and show them how to avoid adjustment pitfalls in the wake of their losses. Finally, explain that the book (Lesson 8) will provide information about finding and accessing supportive resources.

Normal Feelings After Losing Functions and Skills

Reassure clients that the experience of disability-related loss and changes in one's life can lead to doubts about being able to cope. Explain how the media and periodicals in our culture can further these doubts. Relay the role of "Pop Psychology" and the press in instilling doubts by teaching people to monitor themselves closely for depression and other pathological states following common life events. Emphasize that while it is critical to treat depression when it occurs, it is also important to know that some emotions following brain injury and life events are normal. Remind clients that in earlier times many people viewed their emotions after tragedy—death in the family, loss of businesses, even physical injuries—as normal. It was also considered normal to have intense feelings about these events without making the feeling itself a catastrophe. Point out that people successfully made it through their grieving for the most part. You might ask clients if they have lost someone through death, and how they handled their grief. (Note: If a death occurred at the time of the injury, this may not be a good subject to broach.) Point out that during Christmas and the holidays they may have noticed that newspapers and magazines ask readers to take short quizzes to see if they are depressed. Tell clients that you support the idea that people can grieve a loss without being thought odd or pathological. Invite and provide assistance for clients to complete the questionnaire in Box 4.3 in Lesson 4 of their book.

Tell clients that if they answered "Yes" to at least 60% of the questions in Box 4.3 that the chances are good that they are experiencing the normal range of emotions people have after a brain injury. Explain that loss, of functions and abilities, is a part of the brain injury experience. Tell them that brain injury doctors have asked clients in their rehabilitation programs these same questions and found that most reported normal symptoms of grief in varying degrees of intensity. Explain that the doctors also found that persons with even very new disabilities were on average no more depressed than persons without disabilities. However, the therapist should emphasize that the feelings resulting from injury- or illness-related losses can still be very unpleasant and difficult to deal with and that some folks do develop depression in the face of the challenges of brain injury. Point out that sometimes even doctors have difficulty telling the difference because of overlap in symptoms of anxiety, depression, and normal, expected grief reactions. Call clients' attention to Box 4.4 in the companion book and tell them that this is a list of grief symptoms identified by medical doctors and researchers.

As you help clients read the list in Box 4.4, you should ask clients if they have had any, or even more than one, of these grief symptoms. If they endorse some symptoms of grief on the list, point out the similarities between grief symptoms and symptoms often associated with depression and other emotional disorders. Point out that, as with many things in life, a matter of degree is often what separates normal from pathological. Using the degree concept, explain that people should decide whether they need professional help, and seek it, if their emotional symptoms are severe, and with them most of their waking hours because they may actually be depressed and not simply grieving. Provide an example of a person who thinks about their losses so much that they are unable to do daily tasks or sleep for nights at a time. Go on to explain that having thoughts of suicide would definitely be a warning sign that the person who thinks they might be depressed should seek professional help in adjusting to the changes their brain injury has caused. Call their attention to Box 4.5 in Lesson 4 of their books, and explain that it is a guideline for doctors who diagnose and treat people with depression. The American Psychiatric Association's *Diagnostic and Statistical Manual-IV-TR*, clearly outlines criteria for diagnosing a person with depression. (The chart in Box 4.5 provides a few examples of the APA criteria, adapted for simpler reading).

Tell clients that if they, or a family member or friend, have concerns about the possibility of depression, it is important to check with their physician or psychologist to be sure. Make sure to emphasize the point that depression, even after a brain injury, is a very treatable disorder.

Introduce and demonstrate some coping ideas and strategies for common but distressing and uncomfortable grief symptoms following brain injury. Using Box 4.6 of the companion book, Lesson 4, talk about some common grief symptoms, emotional reactions, and disruptive behaviors after brain injury and the suggested way of managing the intensity of that symptom. The therapist should spend the most time describing and demonstrating coping ideas for the problems that their clients have specifically reported. Drawing upon your knowledge and expertise with evidence-based interventions for the problem areas featured in Box 4.6, you should take a step-wise approach to building client capacity with each of the appropriate coping ideas listed.

Tell clients that there will be many other coping ideas in the Lessons ahead. Tell them to practice the Lesson 4 techniques that match their identified concerns at least once a day.

Summarize the take-home points of Lesson 4 for clients using this list.

Lesson 4 Take-home Points

- Brain injury results in losses which bring on normal grief feelings and reactions.

- Common symptoms of brain injury include difficulties with attention, memory, reasoning, problem solving, restlessness, mood and coping, behavioral control, sleep cycles, swallowing, sensory perception, and muscle strength and control.

- Common symptoms of grief include longing for what was lost, feeling sad about what was lost, wishing for the time before the injury, and being upset by reminders of what was lost.

- Everyone grieves in their own way, and length of time varies from person to person.

- People recovering from disabling injuries and illnesses are, in general, no more likely to be depressed than persons without disabilities. If they do become depressed, the disorder is one of the easiest to treat.

- Not only persons with brain injury, but also their families, friends, and others who care for them may experience a sense of loss.

- There are many healthy and productive ways to go through the grieving process and successfully recover emotionally from brain injury.

- Several coping strategies have proven helpful for persons adjusting to brain injury including positive self-talk, keeping active, and proactive self-management for preventing excessive fatigue and depression.

State for clients that Lesson 4, and the Lessons that follow in the book, will give them many additional ingredients for a coping and emotional recovery plan. Explain that all the Lessons will provide clear information and ideas to help them navigate through the challenges of brain injury, deal with losses in healthy ways, and move toward strength and renewed interest in living with disability. Explain that all Lessons will have worksheet sections and questionnaires with instructions as well as summary sections to help them remember the main ideas presented.

Summary

Summarize for clients that disabilities resulting from brain injury are like ripples in a pond when you are trying to skip stones. From that one event, ripples keep moving outward, touching all aspects of a life. The stone hits the water—the injury happens—and the effects spread out over time and relationships. A person can easily feel overwhelmed, sad, confused, afraid, grief-stricken, and defeated. Everyone reacts differently to changes in how they act, look, speak, eat, eliminate, feel, and think. Each person's injury is different. Every person's recovery has a different time frame and course. Mention that there are many different ways an injury can affect each person's day-to-day functioning and the people within their social network. The potential for them, their friends, and their family members, to have a range of fluctuating feelings of various intensities, exists throughout the recovery period and beyond. Recommend to clients that the consistent use of the strategic coping methods and techniques outlined in Lesson 4 will be their best help for overcoming these common challenges and for moving forward in recovery.

Lesson 5 *Anger, Guilt, Acceptance, Denial, and Behavior*

Overview

In the preceding Lesson, you taught persons with brain injury about patterns of thinking that make coping difficult. In this Lesson, the intent is to instruct persons with brain injury about specific common emotional responses to having a brain injury. There are three major ideas that you will want to communicate:

1. There are cognitive underpinnings for emotions, particularly guilt and anger.

2. Persons with brain injury *can* emotionally respond to brain injury effectively.

3. Persons with brain injury can achieve "acceptance."

Rationale

1. Many persons with brain injury are trapped by guilt or anger. The guilt is self-directed around issues such as the cause of their brain injuries (driving too fast, being intoxicated, etc.) or life decisions prior to onset that were destructive (alcoholism, estrangement from family, dropping out of school, etc.). Their anger is typically directed at others either for causing their injuries (being hit by someone else, negligence by someone at work, etc.) or for actions after their onset (poor care, poor legal representation, divorce, etc.).

2. It is usually very difficult for persons with brain injury to move on in life with such emotions because they represent looking backward to past choices by others or themselves.

3. Since the consequences of brain injury are so great, it is very difficult for persons with brain injury to determine how to re-conceptualize their emotions. Absent re-conceptualization of their feelings, they become stuck in anger and guilt.

4. Explaining that anger and guilt are the result of thoughts provides a framework for persons with brain injury to see that they can choose how to view their injuries. It puts them in control of their emotions. Otherwise, the emotions of anger or guilt destructively paralyze them.

5. Being in control is an important concept for persons with brain injury since brain injury tends to remove their sense of self-efficacy.

6. Once anger and guilt are addressed, acceptance becomes possible.

7. Most persons with brain injury misunderstand acceptance and resent those who tell them to accept their injuries and move on with life.

8. Providing persons with brain injury with a format for rethinking acceptance is crucial.

Presenting the Goals of This Lesson

It is important to make sure at the start of this Lesson that persons with brain injury appreciate that they can make emotional changes and that they are not victims of emotional forces that are beyond their ability to understand. Often persons with brain injury may say that they cannot do anything about their feelings; they may say "It is just how I feel," as if the feelings are imposed by some outside force. Providing confidence to the persons with brain injury is important at the start of this Lesson.

Review the following goals of this Lesson with clients.

- To learn what causes both anger and guilt

- To make it easier to reach acceptance

- To realize the destructive nature of denial
- To avoid living in the past

Again, communicate how achievable these are.

Addressing Common Responses to Having a Brain Injury

Persons with brain injury may be surprised to learn that their thoughts about their injuries are shared by other persons with brain injury. Ask them to read the following list and comment on whether they sound familiar. See if they have other thoughts that would fit the common themes of anger or guilt.

"Why did this happen to me?"

"I can't believe I will ever be happy again."

"Life is over."

"I want to find the person who hit me."

"Leave me alone. I don't want your stupid therapies."

"I feel so guilty that I caused my accident."

"I feel like I am being treated like a child again."

Communicate that these are common responses and are normal. People, when faced with as dramatic a change as brain injury, feel overwhelmed and are flooded with primal emotional reactions. Make sure they know that these emotions can be seen early after injury, but can persist for a long time after the injury.

Teaching a Common Basis for Anger and Guilt

As we know, people tend to think of emotions and thinking separately without awareness of how one influences the other. The challenge of this section is make persons with brain injury aware of how their thoughts drive their feelings.

One challenge you may encounter is that persons with brain injury may not be able to identify their feelings. You may find it helpful to digress from their book momentarily and explain how to identify feelings. You can explain that feeling words are usually one word – angry, happy, satisfied, contented, etc.—whereas thoughts are usually sentences—"I think that is a good idea." This distinction is true even if the sentence uses "I feel…" such as in "I feel that is a good idea." It may also be helpful to instruct them that "good, bad, ok, etc." are not feelings but descriptors of whether they are feeling positive (e.g., happy, pleased, tender) or negative (e.g., depressed, disappointed, angry) emotions; good, bad, ok are not emotions themselves. Finally, it might help to ask them to generate a list of sample emotions that you could supplement if it is too sparse. Persons with brain injury may also have language difficulties that mean they need more support in listing or understanding the meaning of emotional words.

Focusing on the normalcy of anger and guilt is essential to help persons with brain injury feel comfortable discussing their own feelings. Then move onto how **thoughts are the key to emotions**. To do this use the example below. You may want to tell the persons with brain injury that you are going to discuss where emotions come from in general and then will return to guilt and anger specifically.

Tommy as an Example

Suppose Tommy is sitting at his desk late on a Friday and the boss comes in to tell him that he needs to work over the weekend to get a job done. Tommy flashes angry. He remains mad all weekend.

Point out to the persons with brain injury that immediately upon hearing what his boss said, Tommy **thought** how unfair the boss's demand was. He wondered why he was being singled out for more work, particularly since he works so hard. He thought that the boss should not make such a request and was not supposed to require weekend work. Tommy's emotions were in response to these thoughts.

It is vital to note that these types of thoughts flash through people's heads so quickly that they are hardly aware of them.

Next use the example below. Have the persons with brain injury imagine the same event but with Tommy thinking different thoughts:

"Here is my opportunity to shine. I know there is a promotion coming in my department and I have been looking for a chance to stand out. Maybe my boss selected me because he trusts me and wants to give me this last chance to excel so he can put forth my promotion rather than Joe down the hall."

Show the persons with brain injury how these thoughts do not trigger anger. Of course, Tommy might still feel disappointed that his weekend plans have to change, but not anger. Direct the persons with brain injury to see the difference: Tommy's thoughts between the event (of his boss's statements) and his emotional response have changed.

Educate the persons with brain injury that in all situations people emotionally react to their own **thoughts** about an event, **not** the event. Dr. Albert Ellis teaches that it is how they view the event and the actions of others that determine their feelings. This should be explained as empowering: while it is hard to control feelings, they are in charge of their thoughts and those thoughts control their feelings.

Examine How People Usually Relate Events and Feelings

To make it apparent how most people operate, highlight that when people experience emotions they relate the feelings to events. See if the following comments sound familiar to the persons with brain injury:

"My wife made me so mad today."

"I am angry that the boss is making me work late again."

"I feel guilty that I did not clean the house today."

Note for the persons with brain injury that the people saying these things are linking their feelings to the events: what the wife did, what the boss did, or what they themselves failed to do. Help the persons with brain injury to understand that we all attribute our feelings to the actions of others or to our own behavior so often that we fail to realize that we do it. Yet, in doing so we miss a crucial component in understanding where feelings come from.

It may be useful to identify the thoughts you are discussing with the persons with brain injury as "interpretation" of events: When an event happens or someone does something, people interpret it (often instantly) *before* people have emotions.

Show the persons with brain injury the diagram in Box 5.1.

Emphasize that the feelings they experience are in response to their interpretation of the event. This happens so fast they don't even realize that it is happening. Thinking about something differently leads to feeling differently about it because emotions are in response, not to the event, but to our interpretation of the event.

Ask them to keep in mind Box 5.1 and tell them that you are going to apply it to anger and guilt. You may want to remind the persons with brain injury that you are now returning to guilt and anger from the general discussion of emotions, starting first with anger.

Presenting the Emotion of Anger

Ask the persons with brain injury what thoughts they have when they are angry? They may say they don't know or they may struggle to recall them. Reassure them and tell them that actually the list is much shorter than most people realize. If they list some, formulate them in the format of the five general samples below.

Note for them that whenever people are angry it is always because other people did something they did not think the other people should have done or the other people failed to do something they thought the others should do.

Relate that their thoughts will always be one of the following when they are angry:

"They should (or should not) do …"

"They are supposed to (or not supposed to) do …"

"They have to (or have not to) do …"

"They ought to (or ought not) do …"

"They must (or must not) do …"

Recall the story of Tommy who thought the boss "***should not*** make such a request and was ***not supposed to*** require weekend work." If the persons with brain injury cannot recall the example, return to it above and review it with them.

Make sure the persons with brain injury understand these words—"should, suppose to, have to, ought to, and must"—set their expectations for other people. The emotion that follows these thoughts is anger. When people do not follow the clients' expectations, they get angry. Make certain that they understand that every time they are angry, it is because someone else failed to live up to their expectations.

Presenting the Emotion of Guilt

The discussion of guilt follows a similar format to that of anger. The difference is that the persons with brain injury have failed to live up to standards they set for themselves. Tell them that guilt is the emotion they feel when they apply the thoughts listed above to themselves. Help them to see the parallels between the two sets of statements. It might be helpful to write them down side by side. The set for guilt is on the left and the set for anger, reproduced from above, is on the right.

Guilt	**Anger**
"I should (or should not) do …"	"They should (or should not) do …"
"I am supposed to (or not suppose to) do …"	"They are supposed to (or not supposed to) do …"
"I have to (or have not to) do …"	"They have to (or have not to) do …"
"I ought to (or ought not) do …"	"They ought to (or ought not) do …"

"I must (or must not) do …"   "They must (or must not) do …"

The guilt thoughts/interpretations occur when the persons with brain injury fail to live up to their own expectations. The emotion that follows these thoughts is guilt. Highlight that when they do not follow their own expectations for themselves, they feel guilt. It is important for the persons with brain injury to realize that ***every time*** they feel guilty it is because they failed to live up to their own expectations.

To help summarize the preceding information show the persons with brain injury Box 5.2. To make it simple, have them realize that the crucial take-away message is to be on the alert for thoughts that involve the five words in Box 5.2. It may make it simpler when they see that the material you have covered can be boiled down to watchfulness for five words in their thoughts.

The thoughts leading to anger and guilt are listed in Box 5.2 in the companion book.

Okay, now let's apply our understanding of anger and guilt to brain injury.

Applying the Five Words to Brain Injury and Anger or Guilt

By now they are probably wondering what Dr. Ellis's ideas have to do with brain injury. Inquire as to whether there is anything they regret about their injury and the actions they engaged in or the behavior of anyone else. Usually there is considerable disappointment expressed about other people or themselves.

Listen for statements like "The person who hit me ***should*** have been paying better attention when driving" or "My spouse doesn't understand me after my injury and he ***ought to*** do a better job of it" or "My doctor doesn't spend enough time with me and he is ***supposed to*** be more caring."

For guilt, you may hear them say "I ***ought to*** have known to wear a helmet when I went bike riding" or "I was ***supposed to*** be smarter and not drink and drive." Help them to see the expectation these thoughts convey and the emotions that derive from them.

Suggest to them that before looking at what to do about these thoughts that they examine examples from their own life. Instruct them to complete the exercise in the companion book.

After they have written their responses, review them. It may be challenging to draft their thoughts in the "should, supposed to, have to, ought to, and must" framework. They may need help in identifying thoughts that carry these ideas implicitly but not explicitly. For example, they may write "I was angry because my son did not clean his room" and "He knows that this is his responsibility" with the implicit "and he knows he is supposed to." Help the persons with brain injury identify the implicit, making it explicit.

Introduce What To Do About Thoughts that Lead to Anger and Guilt

To encourage the persons with brain injury that they can change these thoughts, it can help them to understand where these originated. Most of these expectations were learned when they were young from parents, teachers, television, or other kids. They accepted them since they did not know whether or not they were good standards. In fact, as children they were not allowed to choose their standards: "You will make your bed every day." This was not very negotiable as a little kid. Of course, they were not held very responsible. Nothing really bad happened if they didn't make their beds (although it may have seemed that way at the time).

As teenagers they began to have some freedom to set their own standards: "You should be home by 10 p.m." "Can't I stay out until 10:30 p.m.?" "Okay, but you had better show you can handle it and be on time or you will be grounded forever." They had some say and the penalties went up. Another example with more significant consequences might have been, "All right don't study, but you won't get into college." When they were teenagers they began to understand the link between choices and real-world responsibilities.

It is important to review the proceeding ideas with persons with brain injury. Typically they assume that the way they were taught has to be the way they live. Sometimes there are better choices. If they fail to realize that they live by standards chosen by other people, they are stuck with programming from childhood. Teach them that as adults they get to decide what standards they want and are responsible for the consequences. If they don't want to make their bed, it is okay, as long as they don't mind the mess. However, a messy bed may be less important than sleeping longer and not having time to make it. If they choose to pay bills late, it is okay, as long as they don't mind affecting their credit rating, but timing payment to help cash flow may be more crucial. If they do not work hard, they will probably not get promoted or get a raise, but recreational time maybe more valuable then working extra hours.

You can use Box 5.3 in the companion book to show them the relationship between freedom to choose and responsibility at different life stages. The idea is that as adults they are freer than any other time in their life to select how they want to be.

Prepare Them To Choose Their Thoughts

Highlight that the problem is most adults don't choose. They continue to live according to expectations they learned a long time ago. What they believe is proper is often what they learned as a child, but now those standards may be interfering with their happiness after brain injury.

You can use the following examples to show them how this works. "Good people work" translates as "I am **supposed to** be employed," implying that they are a failure if they are not working. *But* they really know they lost their job because of their injury, not because they don't want to work. "Achieve independence" translates as "I **should not** need help with mobility, managing my finances, and making decisions," implying that they are less worthwhile if they need help. *But* they really know that people with medical conditions sometimes do need assistance. "Pay attention and be reliable" translates as "To show people I am competent, I **ought to** attend to details and complete tasks on time," implying that they are useless if they do not manage their time and cognitively process well. *But* they really know that their medical condition causes these, just like someone who loses a leg has trouble walking.

If the persons with brain injury are having difficulty seeing how these statements lead to guilt or anger, the first example from above about working is outlined in Box 5.4 in the clients' book. Reviewing it with them may help. You could diagram each example above for them similarly.

It is a good idea to discuss with the persons with brain injury their perspectives on the phrases after the "*but*" in each example from above. To the degree that they agree about the reasonableness of each "*but*," they can realize the **unreasonableness** of the expectation that leads to guilt or anger.

Showing the persons with brain injury that low self-esteem stems from their thinking is a crucial link for you to make for them. The proceeding examples were chosen to demonstrate how easy it is to feel worthless and useless if they base their emotions on thoughts learned a long time ago. Instead, as an adult they can change how they view events by changing the thoughts that dictate their emotions.

Having Them Choose Their Thoughts

Have the persons with brain injury look at the following example of changing the thoughts from Box 5.4. Ask them to change their thinking. If they struggle to do so, relate the following change for the thoughts in Box 5.4, changing those thoughts to: "I'd prefer to work, but I can still feel good about myself if I don't work. I can do other things such as being a peer counselor, volunteering, serving on a government committee on brain injury, helping to lobby my legislature on laws about brain injury, serving on a hospital citizens' committee, etc." This change is presented, too, in Box 5.5 in the companion book. Have them compare their suggested change, or the one in Box 5.5, to Box 5.4. Another positive thought might be: "I am contributing to society by spending more time with my kids."

Hopefully, they can see how rethinking things changes how they feel. Guilt is replaced by hope, satisfaction, or pride in this example.

Work with the persons with brain injury on other practice examples. Have them try changing:

"I need help with mobility, managing my finances, and making decisions and I shouldn't need help with those." Or work together on this one: "I am not good at details and time management but I'm a grown-up, and I'm supposed to be good at it." Those thoughts can be reworked; if they cannot determine how, then review the following changes:

- "Yes, I need help with mobility, managing my finances, and making decisions, but I use that as an opportunity. I can teach others about how to help people with needs similar to my own. This can be a two-way street with my getting the help I need in exchange for teaching my providers the best way to help people."

- "I am not good at details and time management now. Instead I will look for opportunities to help people see the brain injury picture. Too many people get lost in the daily grind of details to have long-term vision. Plus, working on thinking about the brain injury picture often is less time dependent than solving the immediate crisis."

At this point it is useful to use examples that the persons with brain injury generate. Have the persons with brain injury return to the example of anger and complete the exercise in the companion book.

Help the persons with brain injury to make the link between new thoughts and decreased anger and guilt. Discuss with them how they might have felt differently at the time if they had thought about the situation in an alternative manner.

Reviewing Why Removing Anger and Guilt Is Crucial

They may question why removing guilt and anger is so important. After all, what is so much better about disappointment compared to anger, or dissatisfaction compared to guilt? The answer that helps many persons with brain injury is that guilt and anger are so destructive. Decreasing anger and guilt is healthy. Guilt and anger increase stress; however, disappointment, dissatisfaction, or other emotions let them make more reasoned judgments and create in them the freedom to problem solve, learn from experience, and to forgive themselves or others.

Applying This Lesson Next Time

There are a few steps to make it easier for them to apply this Lesson in the real world. Review with them the following:

- Every time they think a thought using "should, suppose to, have to, ought to, or must," have them write down the thought.

- Ask them to think about where they learned that standard for their own behavior or the behavior of someone else. Who taught them that thought?

- Instruct them to reflect now as an adult about whether they think that it is a good, healthy, reasonable thought, standard, or expectation for them. Is it making them happier, more content, less angry, or less guilty?

- If it is harmful to them, tell them that now is the time to change it. They can choose; they do not have to live their lives by outdated thoughts that no longer apply to them.

It is often also instructive to have them write down every time someone else tells them that they "should, supposed to, have to, ought to, or must" do something, or not do something. All day long people will lay their expectations on them. They will probably be amazed at how often other people want them to act in a certain way and hope they feel guilty if they do not act as others wish them to do.

Box 5.6 in the companion book can be copied and used as a log of their anger- or guilt-producing thoughts (arising from themselves or other people) and the alternative thoughts that make them feel better.

Helping with the Next Step: Acceptance

While decreasing guilt and anger are fine goals, for most persons with brain injury there is a bigger hurdle. If they can let go of their old thoughts, they are now ready to consider acceptance of their injury. What trips up most people is the belief that acceptance involves no longer letting the injury upset them. When someone says to them that, "You have to accept the injury and get on with your life," it implies the other person believes that the persons with brain injury should no longer worry about their brain injury or be bothered by it.

It will help the persons with brain injury to know that you think that is unrealistic. It can even be irritating when people imply that they quit worrying about it. If the persons with brain injury believe that acceptance means, "be fine with your injury," they will find it very hard to achieve acceptance.

Teaching How Acceptance Can Really Work

It is essential that you provide the persons with brain injury an alternative type of acceptance. The alternative, *achievable* type of acceptance sounds like this: "I hate my injury. If I had one wish it would be to wish it away. **But**, it is not going away because I don't like it. So, I can have strong negative emotions about the injury and still do the best I can. I do not have to be happy about the injury to no longer dwell on it." Fortunately, this kind of acceptance is achievable. In fact, most people who are successful in their emotional outlook after injury achieve this type of acceptance.

The challenge is be able to hold in their mind and heart two separate ideas: "This is bad; I can have a good life anyway and be at peace." The hard part is holding onto two seemingly conflicting ideas: "I don't like this" and "It isn't going to stop me." Note for them, however, that nowhere in those two thoughts is "It doesn't bother me." Rather, they do not have to be frozen in place by their dislike of the brain injury.

For many persons with brain injury it will be a relief to learn that acceptance does not mean having to be Okay with their injury. Many persons with brain injury are distressed inside when people keep telling them to "accept it and learn to live with it." The new perspective on acceptance is often refreshing and invigorating. To achieve this acceptance, they can still regret the injury. They can even be mad about it, if they choose. They can miss the life they had before the injury. **But**, the injury is not all there is to know about them and it is not their total life. They can achieve, love, fail, succeed, hope, etc., even with the injury. Life awaits them.

To get persons with brain injury starting on acceptance have them complete the exercise in the companion book.

Talk with them about realizing that they can still have those thoughts, if they want, but that they can get on with their lives. There is nothing about those thoughts that has to stop them from participating in the best lives they can build.

To begin, have them tell you how they think of themselves and their brain injury. Do they think of themselves as a "brain-injured person," or do they think "I am brain injured?" Suggest instead they begin to think of themselves as a "person with a brain injury." This changes the focus from the injury being all someone would need to know about them. When they change their view to the brain injury being one thing about them, along with lots of other things, some of which they like and some of which they do not like, they open up possibilities for their lives. When they accept their brain injury in this manner, it becomes something to deal with, not something to freeze them in place. They don't have to like their injury to be happy with their lives.

People who achieve acceptance after brain injury view their injuries as an important part of them, but it is not the only part of them. They find acceptance through looking at their whole self. The brain injury does not remove their capacity to have accomplishments, relationships, disappointments, dreams, etc.

Acceptance is difficult if they view their injury as all encompassing. It is achievable, if they view it as part of them, but only a part.

The most crucial message to convey is:

> **THE BRAIN INJURY IS ONLY A PART OF YOU.**
>
> **YOU ARE A *PERSON* WITH A BRAIN INJURY,
> NOT A BRAIN-INJURED PERSON!**

Linking Identity with Acceptance

The intent of the previous section was to facilitate for persons with brain injury the feeling that they are valuable and important. Once there is acceptance of the injury, the next step is to address self-identity.

Most persons with brain injury want to be "independent." However, independence is a myth. Teach the persons with brain injury that we tell ourselves that we are independent so that we can feel secure, and that we do so because it comforts us to think that we could survive alone. After brain injury they have learned that they need other people, but they may not realize that so does everyone else. We all rely on one another.

They are ahead of the game because they know that they need other people. True independence comes not from being able to act alone, but from being so well enmeshed with other people that everyone feels valued and safe.

Make explicit for the persons with brain injury that the issues they must address are often based in society's limited view. Dr. Rhoda Olkin writes that having a disability makes them part of a minority group. It is the only disability group one can join. People join through brain injury, spinal cord injury, polio, diabetes, etc. It is the largest minority group in the country. If you can help them conceptualize themselves now as part of a minority group, their approach to life can change. Minority groups add strength to society.

To help them understand this, have them step back from brain injury for a moment and look at four examples.

Case Examples

Imagine all of the trees in a forest are the same kind (e.g., elm trees). An insect attacks the forest and likes elm trees in particular, destroying all of them. It wipes out the forest. Instead, if some trees were elms and some were oaks and some were pine trees, the forest would survive. Diversity is crucial.

Consider a football team that has too many wide receivers and lineman but only two running backs. When both get hurt there is no one to fill in and the team does poorly having to rely on throwing the ball too much. The team suffers because it lacked diversity. In football, you need lineman, safeties, quarterbacks and running backs, all with different skills.

Think about a so-called individual sport like tennis. If the tennis player had to truly operate alone the player would do poorly. Why? Because the player needs coaches, agents, and trainers with different knowledge and skills. There is no such thing as an individual alone in sport, though we like to pretend there is.

Finally look at work. The best performing workplaces have people with different perspectives. Most of us have been with people who came up with an idea we would not have thought of because of their unique life experiences, training, etc. When companies become too narrow in their thinking (group think) they fail to see market threats and get left behind when things change. Diversity protects us; so-called independence does not.

Being like everyone else is not a strength. Tell the persons with brain injury that they have a unique contribution to make to any group they join. Their experiences add diversity, and it is that richness that is valuable to help others. Just like any minority group member, they can act like their minority membership is an asset or a limitation.

To emphasize this point have the persons with brain injury complete the exercise in the companion book.

Explain to the persons with brain injury that it is also important to realize that their "limits" are more likely a reflection of society than they are of them. Dr. Al Condeluci teaches that we are all "interdependent."

The idea is that when people encounter limitations they attribute these to themselves rather than to how society functions. This is a mistake. This can be highlighted by reviewing the following case example.

Tammy as an Example

Tammy cannot walk and is in a wheelchair. She cannot get into an inaccessible building. She feels it is her problem for not being able to walk. People have said to her she cannot do office work because she lacks the skill to walk around the inaccessible space.

Is the problem one of walking (and therefore her problem) or one of building design (and therefore the employer's problem who loses a great worker)? It depends on how we define the "disability." Maybe the problem is a "disabled building" that does not facilitate access! Maybe instead of saying she has a disability we should say the employer has a dysfunctional building and that she is perfectly fine?

After brain injury, interdependence argues that if we value people's contributions, as we should, then all of us should provide support for that contribution and identify the barriers (cognitive, emotional, behavioral, physical, etc.) that interfere.

Addressing the Issue of Denial

Make clear to the persons with brain injury that acceptance does not mean denying problems. They still must know the issues they have to deal with to move forward. There are two kinds of denial after brain injury[1]:

- Psychological denial

- Organic denial

---

[1] The topic of lowered awareness and acknowledgment of deficit after acquired brain injury is very complex. The following is not intended as a comprehensive discourse, but rather a clinically useful heuristic distinction to guide persons with brain injury. Interested clinicians can pursue further reading with some of the references listed at the back of the book.

Psychological Denial

Explain to the persons with brain injury that the first type, psychological denial, is actually common to most people. It can occur in regard to brain injury or anything else that is hard to face. *Psychological denial occurs when something is too painful for people to admit as being true about them.* It represents something that they find so painful to acknowledge that they reject its validity. If they have psychological denial about their injury, or its fallout, then it is likely that the injury has affected their core beliefs about who they are and how they valued themselves. This is frequently true after brain injury and is normal. After all, they have been through a dramatic shift in their abilities and may feel their self-concept has been under attack.

In such situations it is usual to see a self-protective response involving psychological denial. If they can ignore some of the problems they are having, then it will be easier to hang onto their core beliefs—financial stability, independence, good looks, athletic prowess, intelligence, etc.,—about who they are. Still, with psychological denial they know what the truth is, it just hurts to admit it.

Use the following example to delineate this for persons with brain injury.

Case Example of Psychological Denial

Tommy wants to get back to work. He insists he is ready to his health care workers. When his wife expresses concerns about his balance, he gets angry at her. He even tries to walk close to walls or stay at the back of a group of friends when walking so they cannot see if he stumbles. He purposefully leaves his cane at home when he goes out.

However, in his heart he knows he is less steady than before his injury. He is very fearful of not being able to go back to his own job. When he insists that he can do so, he hopes everyone believes him. He is really seeking someone who will validate his statements that he can work so that he can feel reassured. He is terrified of the consequences of not working and that people will think less of him. However, he is very concerned that balance problems will get in the way of his job.

Emphasize that Tommy knows he has a balance issue. It is just so scary to admit it because it has large implications for him about who he is as a breadwinner and a man. He is doing everything he can to avoid the truth he knows. This is psychological denial.

Ask the persons with brain injury if they can think of a time when they knew something to be so, but it was too painful to admit. Did they avoid thinking about what they knew to be true? Did they tell themselves things that would disprove what they suspected was true so that they felt better? Ask if maybe they are still telling themselves these things and have not yet been honest with themselves. Relate that confronting the truth can be painful; they can no longer hide behind the story they have told themselves. Still, if they are honest with themselves, they will be more effective in life. It is impossible to be their best when their actions are based on falsehoods they generate to protect themselves from reality.

Have them try the exercise in the companion book to practice addressing denial.

Organic Denial

You should next address organic denial (anosognosia). This may prove more difficult. It is different and is only seen among people who have had brain injury. *In organic denial persons with brain injury are unaware of the problems,* in contrast to psychological denial where they are aware but do not confront the problems. Because the brain is injured and it is the examining tool, when it looks at itself to see how it is doing it adds up the data wrong and concludes it is fine.

To help the persons with brain injury understand organic denial use the following example.

Case example of organic denial

Jeannie believes her memory is fine after her injury. Other people have pointed out to her that she forgets things a lot now but she does not believe them. In fact, she got very upset with a friend the last time this happened. Her friend mentioned to her that she missed their lunch date in spite of his having called the day before to remind her, but she denied that he had called. She accused him of lying to make himself look good and to make her look foolish. She said to him that maybe he was making up his so-called reminder call so that he could blame her for not coming and drop her as a friend.

Explain to the persons with brain injury that if one has memory problems, the brain forgets when it forgot something; it thinks it is doing fine. When their brain tells them something entirely different from what everyone else tells them, and then they *refuse to even consider* that maybe these other people know something the persons with brain injury don't see, they are experiencing organic denial.

This only happens after brain injury. If they did not have a brain injury, but, for example, had a broken leg, their brain would correctly see the facts—inability to walk, leg pain, bone sticking out through the skin, lots of blood—and correctly conclude: "my leg is broken." In contrast, when the brain is injured, it examines *itself* after brain injury, it adds up all the "known" facts, and it gives them the wrong answer!

Organic denial is very hard for people to address because the brain insists it is right. Inquire of the persons with brain injury whether they can recall a time since their injury when other people, who they normally would have trusted, gave them feedback or disagreed with them and they fought with them, ignored them, or insisted that they were wrong. Did the persons with brain injury consider the information the other people had? Were the persons with brain injury 100% certain these other people were wrong? Were they willing to explore the other's idea?

Have the persons with brain injury try the exercise in the companion book to help them gain insight into organic denial.

Explaining Why Addressing Denial Is Crucial for Acceptance

Discuss with the persons with brain injury that acceptance includes dealing with both psychological denial and organic denial. If they want to succeed, they cannot ignore their injury. If they have cognitive processing problems, for example, and they deny (either type of denial) their existence, they will have difficulty being successful. The rest of the world will see the errors they make and will take into consideration their real abilities on a given task, not the abilities they want to have (psychological denial) or the skills they think they have (organic denial). The real world judges on performance. To accept their injury means being honest with themselves. Denial gets in the way of that. It is very difficult to achieve anything in life if they do not know their own strengths and weaknesses.

Go through the following information with the persons with brain injury linking achievement of acceptance and success to decreasing denial.

Psychological Denial and Acceptance

Tell them that when they address psychological denial by examination of their beliefs about how they were supposed to live, they change their expectations for themselves. If they can be comfortable with different standards, then they can begin to feel less defensiveness about the abilities they have lost. Psychological denial only occurs when they need to live up to a standard. It is better to choose to change the standard than live, unsuccessfully, in denial.

Organic Denial and Acceptance

Organic denial is trickier because at its core they don't realize the truth. Their brain is giving them false information. That can be hard for them to recognize. One person with brain injury once went 17 years insisting that he could do his old job and refused to accept other work, despite feedback from family, friends, professionals, and most importantly his former employer, that he no longer had the skills for his old job, but that there were lots of other jobs for which he did have the skills. He refused for 17 years after his brain injury to work at anything else. It is important to listen to the feedback they get from other people. It is unwise for them to ignore an accumulation of evidence over time.

Preparing Persons with Brain Injury That Awareness Can Increase Grief and Anger

Let the persons with brain injury know that you recognize how challenging this can be. Despite its crucial importance, awareness that underlies acceptance can be hard. As their awareness improves they may actually feel worse. During denial they may feel better than when they confront their injury. Let them know that, in fact, psychologists in rehabilitation centers commonly hear people saying that "as I get better, I feel worse." They may experience increasing distress as they become more insightful about the challenges they face. In some ways they may feel that "ignorance is bliss," and as awareness increases they are angrier and more depressed. Plus, they may gain awareness of their situation before they have the emotional coping skills to deal with their sense of loss. Reassure them that this is normal and working their way through these exercises with you can help.[2]

Letting the Persons with Brain injury Know of a Final Trap To Avoid

Ready the persons with brain injury that acceptance is hard to achieve if they compare their life before and after their injury. Relate the following situation to the persons with brain injury.

Linda as an Example

Imagine Linda is walking on a trail. She reaches a fork in the road. She will have different experiences in life down one path versus the other path. She may meet someone on one path and not the other. Perhaps she falls in love

---

[2] Be aware that persons with brain injury may experience a catastrophic reaction. This occurs when they confront performance failures that they are unable to explain because their impaired abstract conceptual abilities discount brain injury etiology. There arises dissonance between their perceived lowered performance and acceptable self-formulation. When they face reality without adequate coping skills or insight and are incapable of reconceptualizing their self-esteem, a lack of self-actualization can occur. They may mask their concerns or they may become aggressive, overwhelmed, or passive. Interested clinicians can begin further reading with some of the references at the back of the book.

with that person. However, she also trips badly breaking her leg. Down the other route she might find a lost and injured dog that she rescues. The owner is wealthy and donates a large sum of money to her favorite cause, but she is so distressed over the dog's injuries that she develops trouble sleeping.

Explore with the persons with brain injury that every moment of life things happen that take their life one way or the other. We have all heard of someone who misses an airplane flight that crashes. Consider even smaller events. They get up a little late in the morning and just miss being in the line at the coffee shop and so never meet someone who would have been a wonderful influence in their life. They will never know what wonderful and troublesome things await them on every path. It is impossible to compare the life they have with the life they missed because they don't know what would have happened down the road at each choice point.

If they contrast their current problems with their imagined successes on the other road, they will find that it is impossible to achieve acceptance and they will probably be depressed. There were certainly bad things also likely to happen to them, along with the good, on the other path, but it is hard to conceive of what tragedies (e.g., death of a child, getting a disease, loss of a job, divorce, etc.) might have happened. It is also impossible for them to know yet what tremendous success, great influences, or soaring achievements they will have in their life with brain injury.

Have them look at Figure 5.1 in the companion book. It shows the losing game that many people with brain injury play when they compare their current struggles with their imagined lost future successes. They ignore unknown disasters on their old life course as well as the good things on their current post-onset path.

Have the persons with brain injury think about Figure 5.1 in their book.

If they find it hard to imagine successes, do not let them be frustrated. Some of the best things may not even be known to them during their life. Teachers, for example, shape lives in ways they may never know about: an elementary school teacher who helps a struggling student learn to read and 25 years later the student becomes a doctor. That teacher will never know, but had there been a different, less invested teacher, student might have never learned to read well and so would have quit high school at some point.

Encourage them that the only way to even have a chance of knowing what they will accomplish is to live their current life to the best of their ability and see what happens. They must embrace life, even with the brain injury, if they want to enhance the likelihood of having good things happen. If they are angry or guilty, they will be frozen. Explain that they should not burden themselves with the impossible comparison of lost greatness and current hurdles, ignoring unknown missed disasters and the current potential for wonderful things.

Reflecting on Reaching Acceptance

It is impossible for there to be a comprehensive list of all the ways they think may interfere with getting on with life. Still, a few thoughts are common to many people and can serve as examples for them as to how to proceed. Ask them to consider whether the following thoughts sound familiar to them: "The injury is unfair. No one should have to put up with the fallout of a brain injury. Such things are not supposed to happen to people. One's life ought not to include such harmful injuries. I was supposed to be able to live a more normal life. I have to raise a family. I must earn a living."

Have them look again at the last seven sentences. Every one of those sentences includes a "should, supposed to, have to, ought to, or must." Yet, we know that there are estimated to be 1.4 million traumatic brain injuries every year and about 730,000 people suffer a stroke annually. So, despite the overwhelming evidence that lots of people get hurt, we all think that we are "suppose to be" immune.

Can they see the sequence from event to thought to emotion to nonacceptance? They have a brain injury (event). "I am not supposed to have a brain injury" (thought). "I am angry" (emotion). "I can't believe that this happened to me" (nonacceptance).

Instead, have them try this on for fit. "I have a brain injury (event). Life is risky and lots of people get hurt. I participated fully in life, driving places, playing sports, doing home repair on a ladder, etc., and there was a chance I might get hurt. Plus, I know that my value in life is based on the type of person I am, loving, kind, helpful, etc., not how much money I earn or how good I look, etc., so I know that I can be a great person even with my injury (thought). I am not happy with my injury, but I am participating in life to the best of my ability" (acceptance).

This feels different because of the thoughts. Now obviously those thoughts do not have to be their thoughts. They can think whatever they want. If they choose their thoughts in such a way as to not lead to anger or guilt, they create room for acceptance.

Behavioral Symptoms of Nonacceptance

You may have to assist with behavioral symptoms of nonacceptance. Acceptance is hard. It takes a daily effort for the persons with brain injury to keep focused on moving forward and not looking back. Yet, they may find themselves frustrated with the struggle. If this is so for the persons with brain injury you work with, make sure they know that this struggle is normal. In trying to adapt to their new circumstances they may experience strong emotions. Sometimes people after brain injury have difficulty expressing their feelings directly, and this may happen to them.

Expressing feelings can be hard because they must acknowledge having the feeling, overcome hesitancy to disclose the emotion to other people, have the language skills to communicate the feeling, and remember the words to describe emotions. For some persons with brain injury the barriers to addressing their feelings are so high that the feelings are expressed only indirectly through their behavior.

Inquire if they think that they are expressing their emotions through their behavior. Do they act in self-destructive ways because of guilt, anger, grief, etc? Do other people misunderstand their behavior? Do other people attribute their behavior to the wrong emotion—one the person with brain injury is not having? Are people not providing them with the help they would like?

Review for the persons with brain injury that the problem is that indirect expression of emotion through behavior leads to miscommunication. If they use behaviors such as withdrawal, noncompliance, demanding things of other people, etc., they risk being misunderstood by other people.

Bring this into focus for the persons with brain injury by having them do the exercise in the companion book.

Suggest that one problem with not discussing their emotions is that their message may not get through to other people. They might do better with a more direct approach. A second problem with indirectly communicating their emotions through behavior is that other people may decide to step in and take control away from them, if their behavior is dangerous to other people (e.g., hitting, throwing things, or threatening other people), or, if their behavior is dangerous to themselves (e.g., running away, trying suicide, using poor judgment that places them at risk for harm). If their behavior is inappropriate, such as hoarding things, stealing, being sexually inappropriate, being socially inappropriate, then other people will once more curtail their independence.

Summary

Tell the persons with brain injury that achievable acceptance will not remove their sense of grief or loss, nor should it. Grief is part of acceptance. Recall for them that part of achievable acceptance is acknowledging that their brain injury is real. They have gone through a significant event. Accepting its reality while proceeding with their life still means that it is all right to admit to a sense of loss due to the injury. The goal, after all, is not to deny the changes, but to avoid getting frozen in place by them. If they can change the anger and guilt that may freeze them in place, and address their denial, then acceptance comes easier. Grief, however, is part of acceptance.

Lesson 6   Coping—How to Maintain a Healthy Outlook

Overview

The goal of Lesson 6 is to give persons with brain injury, and their family members and caregivers, the tools and knowledge they need to identify and avoid or counteract several self-defeating thinking and attitude pitfalls. The therapist will serve as a guide, teaching clients with brain injury methods for periodic assessment of how they are thinking and feeling about themselves and their situation. Validation and reassurance from the therapist about the often unpleasant, though normal, feelings of grief related to losses and changes will help clients move toward awareness and acceptance. In addition to educating clients about avoidance of self-defeating thought patterns, the therapist will describe and demonstrate a skill designed to improve proactive planning and coping. The process of goal attainment scaling will be demonstrated for the client. These new skills will help the person with brain injury to self-regulate and set doable, realistic goals toward prevention of hopelessness and despair.

Rationale

1. Persons with brain injury and their families often find and report that the changes brought about by brain injury are disturbing and frightening, occasionally leading to depression or alienation of needed caregivers.

2. Identification of self-defeating attitudes and negativity will help the person with the brain injury avoid these potential pitfalls and enhance participation in therapies.

3. Helping the person with a brain injury develop a habit of self-assessment will lead to improvements in self-awareness. The brain injury population is known to have problems in this area.

4. Skills in setting realistic, doable goals will help prevent hopelessness and despair in the recovering person with brain injury.

5. Personal stories involving survivors of brain injury will help the reader with brain injury identify with others who have this injury and sustain interest in reading the other material in the book.

6. Exercises that allow the reader to self-assess will make the information and coping ideas more personal and relevant.

Presenting the Goals of This Lesson

Review the following goals of the Lesson with clients.

- Learn how to self-assess thoughts, judgments, and feelings about yourself and your situation
- Learn about 5 self-defeating thought habits and how to conquer them to improve your recovery
- Learn how to use a process of goal attainment scaling
- Learn ways to prevent hopelessness and despair

How About You?

The early days of recovery after brain injury are often a blur to clients in the hospital. Help the client think back to the early days of recovery. Ask if they can recall experiencing such common early post-injury problems as disturbed sleep-wake cycles, drowsiness and distractions from medications and pain, and an altered sense of time. If they are not able to remember, ask them if others in their family or social network have told them about their early behavior and symptoms. Ask the client when they began to realize that they had experienced a significant, life-changing event or when they started to notice changes in themselves. Did it take them longer to get dressed? Were they having trouble remembering therapists' names and instructions? Could they read their own handwriting? Reassure the client that even remembering these early insights into changes could be alarming and upsetting, and that they probably were alarmed back then as well.

Self-Defeating Thinking Patterns

After directing clients' attention to Box 6.1, explain that rehabilitation providers working with persons following brain injury report that their clients make comments like those in Box 6.1 all too often.

The therapist should comment that these kinds of thoughts reflect some of the feelings discussed in several prior Lessons. Begin to introduce the concepts involved in self-defeating thinking patterns by explaining that the above comments no doubt arose in response to fear and are extremely negative. As an example, state that as discussed in Lesson 4, most survivors of brain injury reach a point where they begin to compare their abilities after injury with those they remember having prior to injury. The comparison is not logical, because the survivor was not challenged before the injury like they are after the injury, but many survivors fall into this trap. Explain that, as presented in Lesson 4, people with brain injury often struggle with acceptance because of illogical comparisons. They can begin to dislike themselves or feel despair. As a result, the very people around them that they rely on for support begin to pull away because they are uncomfortable about the survivor's negativity and grouchiness. Introduce Dale's story.

Dale as Wounded Warrior

Dale was fortunate to survive seven months in Iraq. He was pretty lucky. While he got involved in some fire fights, he endured them all without injury. There were a couple of times on patrol when a bomb exploded, twice throwing him on the ground. However, he was happy to find that he could just get up, brush himself off, and keep going. After the second blast he noticed a few changes. He was grouchy and his sergeant noticed he was forgetting to follow through on tasks. Dale was referred to the base hospital for evaluation when these symptoms got worse, and he started arguing with other soldiers to the point of causing fist fights. After a brief examination, he was transferred to the major Army hospital in Langstuhl, Germany for an evaluation to rule out a brain injury. By this time Dale started to see that he was having trouble with memory. Even simple day-to-day tasks seemed overwhelming. Then there were the headaches.

Diagnostic testing did reveal that the blasts Dale had been exposed to during combat episodes resulted in two small bleeds within his brain. The neurologist did not think surgery was necessary but the rehabilitation team recommended he have rehabilitation. Then there was the post-traumatic stress disorder that resulted in Dale seeing some horrible scenes from combat over and over again. He was having bad dreams and trouble sleeping. Dale's wife and children were able to join him in Germany. He was so happy to see them, but was embarrassed to have them see him unable to remember events and things said to him on a day-to-day basis. He began to tell himself he was worthless, damaged beyond repair. His wife and parents tried to encourage him, but he snapped at them and often refused to make an effort during his rehabilitation therapies.

After three weeks he began making very slow progress and could finally be persuaded to really work in therapies. He met a psychologist at the veteran's hospital who helped him begin talking through his terrible memories of his war experiences. At first it was hard to talk about these memories. After awhile he looked forward to having this place to talk openly about his feelings and concerns. Dale's wife was supporting and encouraging him, but he remained irritable and unsympathetic to her issues. She did have their two children to take care of and felt really alone with this. His in-laws moved closer to help the family. Dale got an honorable discharge from the Army. He was not able to get a civilian job. Most days he watched television in his bedroom. He was able to continue his therapies at a local Veteran's Administration hospital. Dale told himself that he was useless and there was no point in trying to look for work or work on his relationship with his wife. Unfortunately, his marriage did not last.

Help clients see how some of Dale's adjustment problems may have been related to his inner thoughts and self-defeating behaviors. If the client is a veteran, especially of the Operation Enduring Freedom or Operation Iraqi Freedoms.

Point out Lesson 4 content related to the need for self-acceptance of brain injury deficits and to avoid a trap of negative comparisons with pre-injury abilities. Assist the client in exploring additional pitfalls of thinking to avoid. Therapists should present the rationale that outlook and coping style adopted both in the beginning of and during ongoing recovery from brain injury affect motivation, the amount of energy put toward rehabilitation, the emotions and emotional health of family, and how well clients recover. Point out that negative outlooks are not always obvious or easy to identify, especially by the person with the brain injury. Tell clients that persons with brain injury, because of their common thinking and problem-solving difficulties, may need help to avoid pitfalls.

Introduce clients to the "Attitude Makeover Questionnaire" in Box 6.2 as a preparation for teaching them how to use the cognitive behavioral strategy of positive self-talk and self-appraisal. Explain to them that the new strategies will help them counteract tendencies to think about the worst possible outcomes and aspects of their situation. State that a first step in learning to manage strong worries and feelings, thus to improve your outlook, is to really understand how you think and feel about your situation. Instruct them to take the survey to learn about their overall outlook and self-view.

Guide clients to notice that some statements on the questionnaire are boldface. Explain that the bold statements are negative comments. Reassure them that if they checked mostly bold statements or wrote some negative comments about their current skills, some of the coping ideas in Lesson 6 may help them change to a more positive outlook. Indicate that clients may learn that they are a primary cause of their own misery. If this is true, explain that changing what they say to themselves will be a key to feeling better. Tell clients that both checking italic or positive items on the questionnaire and writing positive comments about their abilities indicates that they have a positive outlook.

Reassure them that continuing to focus on more positives now and in their future recovery will serve them well through the continuing challenges they may face. Explain that regardless of the items they checked, they will likely find the next pages helpful for learning how to be more caring and kind to themselves as they heal from their injury. They will be learning strategies to help improve their attitude toward themselves and recovery.

Now have clients complete the exercise in Box 6.3 of their book. Assist them by writing their answers for them if they are unable. Explain that the "What Are You Saying to Yourself?" exercise will help them identify whether they are making negative comments to themselves and risking harm to their confidence and recovery. Encourage them to adopt all the suggested strategies to help improve their attitude toward themselves and recovery.

Introduce specific thinking habits and pitfalls, "Outlook Pitfalls," that can worsen clients' self-view, dampen their hopes for their future, and interfere with their progress. Assist clients in reading through each of the pitfalls in thinking and the stories that illustrate the consequences of each negative thought habit. Direct clients' attention to the first of the five Pitfalls in Box 6.4.

Next, help clients read over the comments in Box 6.5, and complete the form in Box 6.6. Ask them if they think they are saying any of these comments of Box 6.5 to themselves. If yes, have them write these down in Box 6.6.

Have them acknowledge how far they have come since the first day they were injured. Introduce the "Consider Joe's Approach" vignette below.

Consider Joe's Approach

Joe was thinking about returning to work. His brain injury rehabilitation outpatient therapists and vocational counselors were encouraging him to begin applying for food service jobs. Prior to injury Joe had been a junior manager for a fast food restaurant. Joe told his counselors "before I was injured, I supervised a staff of six employees. I don't want to make hamburgers in the back. I am not able to walk straight yet, and I feel too tired yet. I will wait until I improve and then apply for my old job." Joe had a severe brain injury when a deer hit his service truck. He had made excellent progress since his injury, but continued to have memory, balance, and vision problems. His counselors were recommending that, because of his great progress, his current strengths could result in a good, solid full-time or part-time job at this entry level. However, rather than take the work, and the increased independence and confidence it might bring him, Joe's comparison with his past self did not allow him to see how much progress it took to get to his current status. He missed an opportunity because he was stuck in a negative comparison with the past.

Tell clients to look at Box 6.7 to learn about the second "Outlook Pitfall."

Next, help the client review *Lorraine's story*.

Let's See What Happened with Lorraine

Lorraine's stroke resulted in her need for a wheelchair, but she gradually improved to the point that she was moving quickly around the brain injury rehabilitation unit where she had been for two weeks. A new client, Gail, was admitted for disabilities after she had a fall and mild brain injury, and the two struck up a friendship. Two days after Gail arrived, Gail's physical therapist told her that she could stop using her wheelchair and switch to a straight cane for walking. Lorraine got upset. She said "Gail has only been here two days and is already walking! I have been in a wheelchair for two weeks and nobody has told me I could get out of it. What's wrong with me?"

Lorraine did not realize that her own progress with speed and skill in using the wheelchair was excellent for her. Lorraine got discouraged because of comparing herself to her friend with a completely different kind of injury. By unfairly comparing herself to Gail, Lorraine undermined her own outlook and did not celebrate her own great accomplishments.

Explain that most persons with brain injury will say they were in bed, maybe unconscious, unable to talk, walk, or do the most basic things on the first day of their injury. State that if asked how much they could do two or more months later, they will describe that they could get around fairly well, talk, at least partially dress themselves, and feed themselves with a regular diet. Now ask clients what they were able to do early in their injury. Ask them to use the first day after injury for their basis of comparison rather than their days before they were injured as a way to feel better. Ask them to acknowledge that they have come a long way.

Ask the clients to read through the items in Exercise C in Box 6.8.

Ask clients to keep the self-defeating thoughts in mind while completing Exercise D in Box 6.9.

Explain to clients that when they only compare themselves with themselves they will be more likely to notice the wonderful progress they have made. They can appreciate their own family's efforts only when they consider their unique situation. Tell clients "The bottom line is: Only when you compare yourself only to yourself, will you truly be able to see, and reward yourself, for your accomplishments. It is always discouraging to try to be someone you are not."

Direct clients' attention to Box 6.10 which describes the third "Outlook Pitfall."

Review the story of Joe. Tell the client that Joe's story is an illustration of the impact of unrealistic expectations on recovery and feelings about progress after brain injury. Explain that while Joe's counselors thought he could get a job, and a job may have improved his quality of life, he held on to his goal of returning to his pre-injury work, work he could no longer do, and refused the new job opportunity. As a result of his unrealistic expectations he lost out.

Guide and assist clients in taking the questionnaire in Box 6.11 to find out how realistic they are at setting goals for recovery. Tell clients that if they checked even a few of the items, Lesson 6 strategies may be helpful for improving their outlook on themselves and their situation.

Introduce Zach's story below by telling the client that clearly most people want to improve their ability to do activities that are challenging for them after brain injury. Add that almost everyone has clear goals for their life and recovery. Point out that goals that are doable help people make progress, feel more confident, and improve the quality of their lives following their brain injury. However, make the point that goals that may be too high can lead people with brain injury toward feeling discouraged and badly about themselves.

Zach's Story

Zach's ATV tipped over and, despite wearing a helmet, he had a brain injury. His hospital recovery and rehabilitation are going well. He is weak on one side so he has to wear a small brace on one calf and walk with a 4-prong cane. Zach is embarrassed when his girlfriend comes to see him. He hates that he walks unsteadily. The Recreational Therapist invited Zach to come on an outing with a group of clients from the Unit, to go to the bowling alley. Zach declined, saying "My goal is to be the same as I was before my injury. I am not going out anywhere until I can walk without a cane and brace!" When Zach went home, he stayed home, back in his room. He started to get really depressed because his goal was keeping him from opportunities to see friends and to get back out doing his favorite activities. If Zach had doable, step-wise goals, he might be out and about instead of sitting in his room.

Introduce the client to the 5-step "Goal-Setting Scale" in Box 6.12. Mention that people can get in a habit of thinking that life has only "the best outcome" and "the worst outcome." Tell clients that for the most part, though, almost everything happens in the middle …. part good, part not so great. Invite the clients to join you in using and demonstrating how to use the Goal-Setting Scale to improve their ability to set reachable and realistic goals. Use the following scenario as a sample for your demonstration: Sara would like to get a job as a receptionist in an office because she was a receptionist before her injury. Her speech is slow and hard to understand as a result of the brain injury so answering the telephone would be a challenge.

Encourage participation by saying "Let's help Sara set a realistic work goal" to clients. Work through each section of the scale starting at the bottom, with "Worst outcome." Ask clients to tell you what they think that would be for Sara. Now go to the top, asking what the "best outcome" would be. Do the "Next best outcome," then the "Next worst outcome," and finally the "Middle outcome."

Point out to clients that Sara now has more than one goal step. Say that even if Sara starts out at the "Next worst outcome" she can continue to advance toward her eventual goal. She will feel good about having work of some kind in the meantime, even if it is not her top choice. That job and social network could lead her closer to her top goal. She has doable goals along the way.

Invite clients to think of a goal of their own. Help them articulate the goal clearly.

Next help clients use the Goal-Scaling Sheet in their book, Box 6.13, to try the strategy with their goal. Ask them to notice that there may be smaller accomplishments they could miss if they just aim for the highest step.

Provide an extra copy of the Goal-Setting Scale. Encourage clients to try scaling another of their goals for practice.

Introduce Pitfall #4 using the material in Box 6.14.

Help clients review Amy's story to show how sneaky awful-izing thinking can be.

Consider Amy's Approach

Amy slipped on some wet leaves as she came home with two bags full of groceries in a heavy downpour. She fell backwards and hit her head. She was diagnosed with a traumatic brain injury. It took about one week for her to begin to come out of the confusion she experienced. Soon she noticed that it was harder for her to talk to others and be understood. She had trouble getting nursing and other staff to understand that she had severe pain in her back and head. Panic began to increase and she started telling herself that "This is terrible. This is the worst thing that has ever happened to me. I don't believe I will recover. I might die."

Amy had trouble sleeping because her thoughts created such intense anxiety for her. A chaplain came by and tried to reassure her that she would get better. She felt like God was against her. She told herself she was a hopeless case. She worried that her husband would leave her.

She worried that she might not be able to do anything. By awful-izing, or always thinking about the worst outcomes possible, Amy put herself in a pit and was unable to see out.

Tell clients that Amy's story shows how the habit of "awful-izing" can take over a person's thinking slowly. Invite clients to try Exercise D to find out if they have a tendency to "awful-ize." Ask them to recall a recent or past event or circumstance that was unpleasant or challenging. Perhaps they had a painful medical procedure, or had a long bus ride only to find out that they had arrived at the wrong spot. Ask them to think back about all the details of the situation. Next ask clients to recall what they were saying to themselves at that time. Explain that the two columns in Box 6.15 labeled "Type 1" and "Type 2" include examples of things that people might say to themselves as they attempt to improve following brain injury.

Ask clients to notice how the Type 1, awful-izing statements are dead ends and lead nowhere. In contrast, discuss with them how Type 2 comments move people toward solutions and proactive coping. Explain that Type 2 comments show what positive thinking can do! Ask clients which column, Type 1 or Type 2, contains statements that sound like what they might be saying to themselves after a difficult circumstance. Explain that if they are in the habit of using more Type 1 statements that they may be guilty of awful-izing, and making themselves miserable. Invite clients to recall a recent challenging experience, one in which they noticed the task was difficult for them to do. Assist them in really filling in as many details as possible. Now help clients use Box 6.16 to fill in the statements they remember making to themselves at the time. When finished, help clients identify their Type 1 and 2 comments.

Next, assist clients in transforming any Type 1 comments into Type 2s and help them write the Type 2s in the second column of Box 6.17.

Suggest that they inwardly transform their Type 1s to Type 2s from now on, assuring them that they will then have a more positive outlook, see a way out of the pit, and feel more in control of their situation.

Introduce Pitfall #5 using the material in Box 6.18. Explain to clients that that the first step, as with the other Pitfalls, is to find out if they are doing this to themselves. Suggest that they monitor themselves on a daily basis. Explain that they should listen to how they treat themselves, what they say to themselves as they go through their day. They should ask themselves, "Am I beating myself up, criticizing myself?" Assist the client in learning how to use the Type 1 and Type 2 chart from Box 6.15, encouraging them to start writing down any negative self-talk in column one, under Type 1 in Box 6.19.

Tell them that just as they transformed their "awful-izing" self-statements earlier, they will now begin to transform their Type 1 self-talk into Type 2. Present the examples in Box 6.20.

Invite clients to continue using this format until they have practiced transforming their negative thoughts into positive self-talk. Note that practice makes perfect!

Summary

Help clients review the discussions and exercises about the several self-defeating habits of thinking that can hinder progress in recovery from brain injury and reduce the quality of post-injury life. Briefly identify and describe all five types: The two self-defeating comparisons, unrealistic expectations, awful-izing, and negative self-talk. Be sure to cover both types of self-defeating comparisons. Remind clients that you talked about these specific pitfalls of thinking, ways to determine if they have them, and ways to reverse them to a more positive outlook and coping. Discuss the strategies they learned for avoiding negativity and discouragement. Tell clients that they are now closer to having the most powerful ingredient for successful healing and survival after a brain injury, a nurturing and positive view of themselves and their ongoing recovery.

Lesson 7 *Thoughts for People in the Lives of Those with Brain Injury*

Overview

This Lesson is written to help you address the concerns of *the people in the lives of those with brain injury*. The exercises are designed for people who have a relationship to a person with a brain injury. The intent of this lesson is to help people other than persons with brain injury, per se.

If you are working with persons with a brain injury who have read the corresponding Lessons in their books, they may find it difficult to read about the stresses and frustrations those significant to them encounter. You might want to discuss with the person with brain injury that this Lesson is very direct about the needs and issues those around them face. Hopefully, if they read this Lesson it will open a sincere dialog with those significant to them.

This Lesson is written for you to act as guide to this material. Still, it recognizes that often there is a team of professionals involved in providing care and therefore, at times, this Lesson also suggests that people talk with other professionals involved in providing care.

Rationale

1. People who know the persons with brain injury are often deeply affected by the injury.

2. Too often, little attention is paid to the struggles of spouses, partners, parents of adult children with brain injuries, parents of young children with brain injuries, adult children of parents with brain injuries, friends, and employers.

3. Most of these people have had no preparation or information before onset about brain injuries and how to respond.

4. They are searching for models of how to handle the life disruption that brain injury entails.

5. They are likely struggling with their own emotional responses to brain injury. The injuries may well have altered their own lives and, yet, they feel guilty about raising such concerns.

6. There is likely hesitancy on their part to ask for help and they may be embarrassed by their need for help.

7. In some cases, despite strong emotional ties to persons with brain injuries, the health care system may dissuade them from being involved with implicit, if not explicit, messages about their involvement.

Presenting the Goals of This Lesson

It is valuable to set the tone of this Lesson with people in the lives of persons with brain injury. Explain that it is normal and acceptable for them to seek help. Indicate that, in fact, it is common and commendable for them to do so. No one handles brain injury in people they care about very well when they try to do so alone.

Review the goals of the Lesson with the people in the lives of persons with brain injury.

- To explain the stresses they may encounter
- To guide spouses/partners, children/parents, friends/employers on handling their unique issues
- To help everyone cope with guilt, frustration, and uncertainty

Again, communicate that it is normal to want and to need guidance about these issues.

Addressing Common Responses by Significant Others

They may be surprised to learn that their thoughts are shared by other people in the lives of persons with brain injury. Ask them to read the following list and comment on whether they sound familiar. See if they have other thoughts that would fit these common themes:

"My wife seems like a different person now and I have to do the work for both of us in our marriage."

"My fiancée doesn't remember me!"

"None of my friends realize how badly hurt my son is."

"My husband can't handle coming to the hospital to see our daughter."

"We are not formally married, but she is my partner and I know her better than her family whose members won't listen to me."

Let them know that, as these sentiments convey, it can be very difficult as a person with a significant relationship to someone with a brain injury to adapt to the demands of life after brain injury. A brain injury in someone they have a relationship with will affect *them*. However, it is likely that they are unprepared for the impact of the brain injury on them and their relationship with the person after a brain injury. This is not surprising.

Tell them that there are three reasons for this:

- Probably no one provided them with education about brain injury before it occurred.

- Each injury is different, so it would be hard to prepare for the changes they are likely to experience.

- The health care system focuses on the care of the person with a brain injury and does a poorer job of attending to the needs of the people who have relationships with persons with brain injury.

So, if they are spouses, partners, parents, children, friends, or employers of the person with a brain injury, they will find a section of this Lesson relevant to them.

Coping for Those in Relationships

The following material is presented according to the relationship people have with the person with brain injury. Use the section most relevant to who you are working with.

Spouses

It is a good idea to let spouses know that family members are often in shock immediately after their loved one has a brain injury. As time passes, shock evolves into being overwhelmed and uncertain. Eventually, a sense of loss develops as their awareness of deficits in the person with a brain injury and changes in their marital lifestyle begin to emerge.

As a spouse, their life is proceeding down a different road than they had planned. In Lesson 5, the normal, but detrimental comparisons the person with a brain injury makes with the life that was lost are explained (see Figure 5.1). As a spouse, they are also likely to make the same comparisons. Hence, it is valuable to review Figure 5.1 with spouses before proceeding further.

You can further explain that there are two reasons why spouses make the false comparison of lost opportunities against current hurdles, ignoring unknown missed disasters and the current potential for wonderful things:

- Little support:
    - They may be receiving little support for the impact of the injury on them.
    - They may feel that they are supposed to focus on the needs of their spouse. If they worry about themselves, they may feel guilty since the role they were taught by our society is to

attend to the needs of the injured person. (See Lesson 5 for how "should, supposed to, ought to, must, and have to" lead to guilt and anger. You may need to review with them some of that material as well.)

- Lost hopes:
  - Their dreams may be threatened by the brain injury.
  - They may have fears about their future.

To start to address their concerns have them try the exercise in the companion book about having too little support. Hopefully they will better understand how their own needs can get pushed aside.

Use their responses to demonstrate for them how easy it is to get trapped into ignoring their own needs and worries. Highlight for them that:

- They may find that their friends, family, and employers may inquire about how their spouse with the brain injury is doing, but forget to check on how they are coping.

- Their usual main source of support during most crises, their spouse, is "unavailable" to them because it is their spouse who had the injury.

- Just as their awareness of the real-world implications of the injury grows over time, their support system of friends and family moves on with their lives and they may experience increasing isolation.

Congratulate them if their support system has helped them over time take care of themselves and meet their own needs. If not, then it is important that they figure out how to decrease their sense of loss and get support for doing so. Let them know that there is hope.

Remind them that it is important that they accept that it is all right for them to be concerned about themselves. The first step is to know what their needs are. Have them look at the checklist in Box 7.1 in the companion book. Have them mark the needs that are currently unmet for them.

Once they have identified their needs, figuring out how to get help and information can seem like a daunting process. Reassure them that there is help and that there are a number of sources of help. First, they can access friends or family members for help. However, the people in the lives of persons with brain injury may need guidance regarding asking for help. Review with them that:

- Friends or family members are much more likely to help than they might first think. The problem other people have is that they assume needs go *down* over time, just like it would if their spouse had broken a leg. Also, if other people are not asked, they assume that things are all right with the people in the lives of persons with brain injury. Most people care and are willing to pitch in to help, if they understand the extent of their needs.

- Asking for help requires that they overcome the hurdle of feeling embarrassed to need help. Remind them that no one is prepared for a brain injury and they ought not to expect that they should be able to handle it alone. It is crucial that they avoid feeling embarrassed for needing help. Embarrassment will stop them from seeking the help that everyone needs after a spouse has a brain injury. To solicit help in the most effective manner, they must be comfortable with self-disclosure.

- They will get the most help when they make their need personal. Instruct them to talk about their feeling overwhelmed and afraid. Tell them to let people know about their sense of loss. Have them be specific, too. If they are at risk for losing their job because they are responsible for transporting their spouse to therapies or a day treatment program every day, teach them to tell their friends that. If they are facing money difficulties, have them see if their friends and family would conduct a fundraiser for them.

- In addition to self-disclosure, they may have to facilitate the education of their friends and family about brain injury. An excellent source of information is their local state chapter of the Brain Injury Association of America or the national organization itself. Some chapters have printed and videotape information. There are usually educational seminars or conferences for spouses, families, and friends. Remind them that in all likelihood other people do not appreciate the implications of brain injury. What knowledge other people have probably comes from misrepresentations perpetrated by erroneous television shows. In those shows, if one blow to the head causes damage, the second blow fixes it!

Second, if they need help and friends or family are unwilling or unable to help, their state Brain Injury Association can often be of assistance.

- Their state Brain Injury Association of America chapter should know who the resources are in their area that help after brain injury. Frequently, there are providers who will help with transportation, respite care, financial planning, etc. You may need to provide assistance and encouragement for them to call their state Brain Injury Association.

- Tell them to ask if their state Brain Injury Association provides case resource facilitation services (a knowledgeable person who can make and coordinate contacts), and if they do, suggest they make the most of them.

Third, they can ask their physician, psychologist, social worker, etc., about who to call for help. As a provider yourself, this may seem obvious, but too many people in the lives of persons with brain injury fail to receive as much resource advice as they might. For example, many are poorly informed by professionals about their state agencies, state Brain Injury Associations, insurance company resources, etc. Moreover, professionals understand how agencies work in ways other people do not. Emphasize that:

- Professionals typically know of services and agencies that provide a wide array of supportive help.

- Professionals can tell them what specific person at an organization, not just the organization, to contact. Quality of service and knowledge about brain injury varies between people at organizations. Also, they will get more personal service when they call someone and say, "I was referred to you personally by so-and-so who told me to ask specifically for you."

- If their provider is recommending that they contact a large organization or system, rather than a person, it may help if the provider makes an initial call for them to assist them in getting through some red tape. Providers sometimes can smooth the way and get a quicker response from organizations. Providers may also better understand what they are being told on the phone and may think of questions to ask on the phone that they would not think to ask.

- It may work best for providers and spouses to make calls together. If spouses and providers cannot coordinate calls together, see if their state Brain Injury Association will facilitate the calls for them.

Recommend that they make a list of what each person they ask for help is being asked to do so that they stay organized. Show them Box 7.2 in the companion book that provides them with a handy reminder form.

Review that there were two reasons why spouses make the false comparison of lost opportunities against current hurdles, ignoring unknown missed disasters and the current potential for wonderful things: little support and lost hopes.

Explain that you will now help them by looking at lost hopes. Suggest that it is all too easy to not even think about their own loss. It is all right to have experienced a sense of loss and they need not have to deny the impact of the injury on themselves. While writing down their losses may seem counterproductive, it may relieve them from living with an ill-defined, pervasive grief that they have difficulty addressing. In the exercise in the companion book see if they can capture their sense of loss.

Provide them with the idea that coping with this sense of loss is a two-step process. First, they must determine whether the losses are real. Many people project the future and assume that goals are out of reach. They have "anticipatory grief" in which they grieve for losses that may not have yet occurred. It would be best to make inquiries of others about how likely it is that the brain injury will cause them to lose a goal they had.

You can advise them to:

- Ask experts in the brain injury field how to achieve their goal and manage the changes imposed by the brain injury. They are likely to find that their situation is similar in at least some ways to scenarios that experts have helped spouses handle previously. The professionals may have ideas, methods, or resources they might not have thought about.

- Ask people involved in their hopes (e.g., for a career goal that they feel is lost, involve their employer) about how they may be able to help them still reach their dream. Many such people will help more than they might imagine if they are asked.

Instruct them to use the form in Box 7.3 in the companion book to write down who they are going to consult with about their hopes.

It is almost taboo to raise the next point, but it bears attention. You should be ready if spouses think about leaving the brain injury behind through divorce. If they introduce this topic, you might prepare to tell them that they are not bad, if they have had thoughts of divorce. When trauma occurs in life and they feel helpless, it is natural to respond by trying to extricate oneself from the situation. However, most spouses begin by wanting to have their marriages succeed in the face of brain injury. This book assumes that they are seeing you to learn how to have their marriage succeed. The challenge is that the roles in their marriage may change:

- Perhaps they are now the main source of income and they may have to begin the act of bill paying.

- Maybe they have to do all of the driving.

- Most of the child rearing may be their responsibility.

You can advise them that to succeed they will need to adjust their expectations for themselves and their spouse. They and their spouse with the brain injury may need to learn new skills. Support them by letting them know that this can be scary. It is all right for them to be worried about how they will do. Remind them that they do not have to do this all alone. Many couples make the necessary adjustment. Learning how to distribute the responsibilities is something they can do, with help, but it takes help.

Be ready with local marriage counseling resources, particularly therapists who understand brain injury, if you or the spouse feel this would help.

Partners

Partners face the same issues that spouses do (and you should have them work through the exercises in the preceding section for spouses), but sometimes with less security, leading to additional concerns. Partners may include boyfriends/girlfriends who have been together a long time, gay and lesbian couples, or people in other relationships.

You should be aware that the lower security arises due to two factors:

- In some instances the lack of clear legal standing causes problems. They may find that their access to information is limited by not having legal standing. In addition, without legal standing they may not be allowed to make decisions for the person with a brain injury. Providers can have their hands tied by legal constraints. Laws and the courts may direct professionals about who to give information to and whose desires to follow for decision making. It is worth discussing these concerns with the providers they are dealing with. They may find there can be some sort of accommodation that can be arranged.

- Other people may respond differently to their relationship than they may hope. Family members of persons with a brain injury may assert their belief in their right to make decisions, rather than partners. They may try to prohibit them from seeing the injured partner, if they disapprove of the relationship. They may try to exclude them from conferences with providers. If there were conflicts in values or if family members rejected the choices their partner had made, the family dynamics surrounding those differences may play out in front of providers.

You should have partners work on the exercise in the book for persons with brain injury. It will help them to consolidate the special hurdles that they have encountered.

The next step is to advise them on how to proceed with their concerns. If their difficulties have been with professionals, then you should direct them to openly raise their concerns with the provider.

- If the providers were unaware of their desires, then the providers should become more inclusive. However, they may encounter some professionals who fail to appreciate their sense of loss and grief, misjudging the emotional impact upon *them* since they may not appear to the providers to have either a traditional or permanent relationship. The professionals may unintentionally disenfranchise their grief. In such cases:

- Have them explain that their experience of grief is heartfelt and true and it is short-sighted to categorize the emotion of loss by the definition of the relationship. Rather, it is the emotional bonds and the personality of the partners that, in part, drive their emotions.

- Tell them to be specific and call attention to their unmet needs. Too often, partners assume professionals perceive their needs. Make sure that they don't rely on such assumptions.

- If the providers are bound by law or regulation, have them ask the professional to give them suggestions on what steps they need to take to become more involved.

- If the professional cannot see a way to help, then advise partners to consult with the facilities' "Patient Advocate" office to see if there is an overlooked solution.

If their issues are with family members, be ready to support them emotionally since it is very difficult to have to address these issues when they are already confronted with their partner's brain injury. Typically partners of persons with a brain injury feel disillusioned, hurt, and angry with family members if those members take actions that seem to deny the partner's emotional ties to the person with a brain injury.

Still, while normal, their resentfulness over having to deal with this is harmful to them. It is likely to make them angrier and less effective. The question is not whether they have grounds for being upset, but whether being upset helps them.

There are three approaches that you can review with them:

- Sometimes partners want to take legal action. This is the most confrontational approach. Sometimes partners seek conservatorship/guardianship in direct opposition to the family. Sometimes the family members respond similarly and then a legal battle ensues regarding who will obtain legal decision-making authority. This can be expensive and time consuming. Furthermore, it is often unclear how successful each party will be in court. You should point out the impact these disputes can have on persons with a brain injury. Advise them that if they wish to pursue this course that the disagreements not be played out *in front of* persons with brain injury because doing so may affect their recovery and coping.

- You should advise them to consider engaging the providers with whom they are working. If as a partner they were significantly involved in the person's life, providers generally want to be able to gather information from as many sources as is feasible and involve all parties, if possible, in care. Providers may be able to help balance competing interests and act as a buffer between estranged partners and family members. A common example occurs when various parties will not communicate, but all will let information flow to providers separately from everyone. They must realize that this works only if the desires of different parties are not diametrically opposed.

- It is worth advising partners that the third recourse is the best: Seek compromise with the other significant people in their partner's life. Too often, people let their own emotional needs take precedence over the needs of persons with a brain injury. See if they can find a way to come together for a common good. Old battles can be fought in the future instead of now. People can be surprised at how well they may work together, if they focus on the problems at hand.

Parents of Adult Children

Parents of adult children with brain injury will present you with unique challenges. The parents of persons with brain injury typically have to confront an array of issues. Often parents feel guilt over their inability to have protected their child from a brain injury. (Guilt of this nature can also occur when the loved one dies.) After all, parents typically consider their first responsibility to be the physical safety of their children.

Brain injury, perhaps the worst damage the body can sustain, rips at people's self-concept as good parents.

Yet, you know that parents generally could not have prevented the brain injury. Most activities that lead to brain injury are usually harmless: driving, sports, etc. Most people do not sustain brain injury in most normal activities. So, it is unreasonable to hold themselves to the standard that they should have predicted a low probability event. Parents are probably not considering the probability of the brain injury, but are just focused on its having happened. You can provide reassurance in the face of their guilt that they could not have predicted the low probability event or prevented its occurrence.

People cannot live continually afraid of everything that *might*, on an off chance, cause an injury. Hence, the guilt they may experience ("If only I had …") is likely unfounded.

To help them, ask them to complete the exercise in the companion book. It helps bring to the forefront the thinking that is leading to their self-blame and makes concrete the advice they have been getting.

Direct them to consider the messages from other people. Perhaps they would feel better if they listened to the messages others are giving them. Let them know that it is all right to be gentle on themselves. Harsh judgment is detrimental to them and to their loved one with a brain injury. Their loved one needs them to be involved in the rehabilitation and recovery process, not paralyzed with guilt. They can serve as a compassionate, but logical resource. Their help is needed. Self-recrimination interferes with effective support.

To cope with their own feelings, parents may fall back into one of two familiar roles in the face of a brain injury crisis: Nurturer or Breadwinner. Yet, both of these roles have pitfalls that you should review with parents.

Roles Issues: Nurturer

One role is resumption of the "nurturing" role they fulfilled when the person with a brain injury was young. This can be a great service. They may be able to provide housing, cooking, transportation, supervision, etc.

They can help absorb some of the burden of care that otherwise might fall on spouses and friends. Still there are risks associated with this role and you want to make sure that they avoid the traps.

- It is easy to burn out if they take on too much of the support load, and if they are feeling guilty, they may well overdo it. Teach them to remember that helping after brain injury is a marathon, not a sprint. They must pace themselves. Fifty percent effort sustained for years is better than 100% effort from which they collapse after six months. (This is true for spouses, too.)

- If they adopt the nurturing role they should be aware that they may be the target for the frustrations of the person with the brain injury. If the role includes setting limits on driving, chemical use, dating, working, independence, cooking, or recreational activities (e.g., snowmobiling, bicycling), they may catch the brunt of the person's anger. Similarly, they may have to enforce compliance with ongoing treatment attendance and recommendations.

- The tendency is for them to revert to the techniques they used as the parent of a young child. However, this is fraught with problems. You must inform them that persons with brain injury revolt against being treated like children. Usually persons with brain injury expect to be treated as they were before their injury.

To avoid these traps, you can discuss the importance of balance. Guide them to provide support, but not to smother. To help them, review these recommendations:

- Seek advice from professionals about what freedoms are permissible and what restrictions are necessary.

- Ask the professionals to take responsibility for promulgating the rules. It is actually best to do this, with both them and their loved one present, so everyone knows that they are following the professionals' advice and everyone has heard the same thing.

- Ask for written restrictions to decrease misunderstandings.

- Look for specific recommendations to implement the restrictions (e.g., to implement the restriction of "no driving" by the person with brain injury, if impulsivity is an issue or the person disagrees about the driving restriction, they might have the specific recommendation to "keep the key with them at all times").

Have them use the form in Box 7.4 in the companion book to record restrictions and specific recommendations.

Make sure that they know that *how* they discuss restrictions with the person with brain injury is essential. Discuss the following suggestions with them:

- Monitor tone of voice and attitude so that it is an adult-to-adult conversation while simultaneously being aware of the person's cognitive deficits (e.g., memory, reasoning, judgment, attention span, insight).

- Avoid being either condescending or angry and frustrated.

- Prepare for conversations. Take time to mentally and emotionally get ready to discuss issues.

Roles Issues: Breadwinner

The other role that parents sometimes re-adopt is that of "breadwinner." Prior to injury, when their adult child was much younger, they provided financial support as the breadwinner of the family. After a loved one has a brain injury, they may find that their most comfortable reaction is to work more. This is a natural response, particularly among parents who are struggling themselves to cope with the injury. Furthermore, since financial distress often accompanies brain injury due to medical bills and loss of employment by the person with the brain injury, it can be extremely important to supplement income. You should make sure that the parent realizes, as with the nurturer role, that the breadwinner role requires balance. Discuss with them the following points:

- Work can be seductive. It can feel safe and familiar in a world that now seems uncertain. Brain injury is an ambiguous loss. Work is something they can control, whereas life after a brain injury seems chaotic.

- They should be careful to avoid withdrawing from their family and their child with a brain injury. It is too much to expect that they will cope well with brain injury when work isolates them.

- If they overinvest in work, their family may perceive them as either doing fine and not needing support or not caring about the stresses on the family. Breadwinners need the emotional support of their families, just as the families need their support.

Roles Issues: Parent of Married Child

There is a final role that is unrelated to previous roles parents may have undertaken. This role can be concurrent with the other roles. If their child is married, or in a relationship, they may need to address the desires of the partner and how all of their roles can complement each other. Too often, conflicts arise between spouses (or partners) and parents about what direction care (e.g., rehabilitation, living arrangements, supervision) should take and how to utilize the resources everyone brings to the situation. You should raise with them how they plan to handle conflicts if they are the parent of a married (partnered) child.

Review with them their feelings about assuming a deferential role when their instincts at seeing their child hurt trigger the previous nurturer or breadwinner roles. They may find themselves wanting to take charge. After all, they obviously have the longest relationship with their child and probably have intervened in the past on their child's behalf. Moreover, they bring maturity and life experience to the situation that spouses or partners may lack. Do not be surprised if they find that they are frustrated in their efforts to impart their expertise and to lead their extended family, if the spouse wants to be in charge.

Of course, the opposite may arise; they may be requested to step in as others flounder and are overwhelmed. This too can be trying, if it is unexpected. If they had accommodated themselves to their children being adults and making their own decisions, it can be jolting to again need to be in charge. Some parents find it difficult to sacrifice the lifestyle they have with their children grown by being drawn into a more intimate, immediate parenting role again, having to cook, clean, drive, etc., for their now adult child. For some parents this is particularly hard if they had a pre-onset difficult relationship with the spouse or partner. They may feel resentfulness or anger in such circumstances. They may even wonder if the spouse or partner will stick with their child through the turmoil of brain injury.

Explain that these are normal feelings. They are not alone in feeling this way. Wanting to take charge, on one hand, or resenting having to do so, on the other hand, are emotions that professionals often see parents wrestling with. Again, advise them to be gentle on themselves for struggling with how to proceed. There is no clear roadmap.

The one thing that really will help is that they be honest with themselves. Inquire as to what they *want* to do? What do they feel *obligated* to do? What can they *handle* doing? Have them work through these questions in the exercise provided in the companion book.

Explain that the answers to these three questions may very well be in conflict with each other. Their desires, responsibilities, and abilities may not match. They may not want to resume a daily parenting role, feel they are supposed to do so, but not feel able to manage it. They may want to be intimately involved, though not feel they have to, but feel capable of it, if needed. These are numerous combinations of answers to the preceding questions.

The best advice you can give them is to seek equilibrium. Have them:

- Discuss their involvement with the professionals working with their loved one. The providers can impart their experiences with previous families as to what is likely to work and what will be ineffective.

- Tell the professionals their feelings and any dilemmas; providers may be able to help them resolve their conflicting desires.

- Make contact through support groups with other parents who are further post-onset who may have valuable insights. (See Lesson 8.)

After they have gathered further perspectives they may decide to be very involved; they may elect to be distantly supportive; or they may select a middle road. Make sure they pick what they believe is best in light of the answers to the three questions discussed above, and what they feel is right for their child. Use Box 7.5 in the companion book for a reminder of the crucial questions for their decision making.

If you are not a therapist for the family, do not hesitate to advise them to ask for therapy with a psychologist for *them*. Implementation of their plan can be stressful whatever answers they settle upon. They may feel that they should be able to independently cope with the impact on them of the brain injury to their child. After all, they probably raised their child without psychological support and, moreover, they are not the one with the injury. This perspective, however, may limit them.

- It deprives them of available support and decreases their access to information about brain injury.

- It feeds into the myth that family members ought to be able to handle chronic medical conditions (e.g., brain injury, spinal cord injury) in loved ones as they do acute health concerns (e.g., a broken bone) without ongoing support.

Have them avail themselves of all the support they can without feeling guilty or inadequate for doing so.

Parents of Young Children

Much of the advice you give to parents of young children is similar to that for parents with adult children (i.e., avoidance of guilt and burnout, getting specific recommendations, going to support groups, and receiving counseling). Nevertheless, there are differences and they may present some unique situations. If they are parents of young children:

- They have the lead role in decision making for young children and they have the role for advocating for the needs of their child.

- They have a long-term commitment to care for their child.

- They must deal with the school system.

- They must contemplate developmental stages and how they will interact with brain injury.

You should be ready to guide parents through these challenges. They may find that their adaptation to brain injury and its accompanying parental lifestyle change is less stable than that of a parent of an adult person with brain injury.

You should prepare them to expect that as children advance through developmental stages, the expression of the brain injury may alter. This provides parents with a continually evolving set of hurdles, requiring different skills from them as their child grows. They must structure different support systems for themselves as their child grows.

For instance, when persons with a brain injury are young, they must be ready to interact with the school system. This is a special challenge because schools vary wildely in their knowledge, attitude, and resources for children with brain injury. In some states, the state agency responsible for education is a wonderful resource. For example, in Minnesota, they sponsor training about brain injury for teachers and others in the school system and prepare written material. Again in Minnesota, there is also a private organization to help parents advocate for educational services (i.e., Parent Advocacy Coalition for Educational Rights at www.pacer.org). In some states they may be surprised to learn, as are many parents, that there may be little help available.

You can advise them to get help from professionals, including:

- Rehabilitation Professional
- School Guidance Counselor
- Special Education Teacher
- School Psychologist
- School Principal
- School District Officer
- County Social Worker
- State Brain Injury Association Chapter
- Private Advocacy Organizations
- State Education Agency

In many cases, parents are unaware of how many resources they can access and how to go about reaching these individuals. You may need to encourage assertiveness to follow up with the professionals listed above. Have them use the form in Box 7.6 in the companion book to list who they will talk to for help.

You may encounter parents who are hesitant to seek help. Society teaches that there should be no burden too great for parents. Those who put forth this idea do so without considering brain injury. Since parents feel an encompassing bond with their children that entails nurturing, instructing, protecting, advocating, etc., and since care post-brain injury in a young child requires so much more of all of these, the burden can become too much.

You may need to teach parents that brain injury exceeds the limits of most people for solo nurturing, instructing, protecting, and advocating. Yet, no one in society puts an asterisk next to parenting children with brain injury. Show them the box below and have them refer to it often.

Remind them often that they will cope better with their grief if they solicit assistance.

PARENTING*

*NORMALLY GIVE IT YOUR ALL,
BUT AFTER BRAIN INJURY GET HELP!

Adult Children of a Parent with a Brain Injury

It is distressful to see a parent injured. Most people think of their parents as a source of support and a solid foundation for life. Many adults struggle to contemplate the sense of loss that accompanies their realization that their parent might be unavailable for sustenance to them. This is particularly true when the loss is abrupt and unexpected, as is typical with brain injury.

You will likely find, in such instances, that three factors come into play that may challenge them:

- They must cope with the shock of the injury.
- They may have to become their parent's decision maker.
- Old relationship issues between them and their parent may resurface.

To address these issues, have them complete the exercise in the companion book, writing down their thoughts about each of these variables.

Examine with them each of these.

First, let them know that it can be gut wrenching to see someone who has been an independent, self-reliant individual now appear so vulnerable and needy. Reassure them that it is all right for them to focus some time on their own sorrow. As they recognize the startling change in their parent, many adult children become weighed down by the emotional trauma to themselves. Instruct them that:

- They are not alone if they are feeling stunned by the changes in their parent, uncertain as to how to reconcile the changes with their image of their parent before onset, and grieving the loss of the relationship they had with their parent.
- They should remember to seek emotional support for themselves. It is easy to fall into the trap of believing that, as an adult, they should be able to cope independently with whatever life throws at them. However, it is very difficult for someone to see a parent suddenly unable to function as before.
- Society offers few role models, little societal support systems, and no training for them to cope with the changes that occur to parents after brain injury. Hence, have them avail themselves of resources through their state Brain Injury Association or their hospital's rehabilitation psychology department for counseling.
- They may also find that a parent's injury causes them to rethink their own values and progress in life. They may even see a parent's injury as a reminder of their own vulnerability. These are profound issues. They relate to the choices they have made in their

life, the successes and regrets they have, and the type of person they are. There are no bigger things to reflect upon in life and they are being confronted with them with no preparation time.

- They ought to be easy on themselves. Do not let them be unfair to themselves by tackling too much emotion at once. Have them give themselves breathing room to process their feelings.

Second, teach them that they may find themselves thrust into the role of decision maker for their parents. This can be very difficult on them. While in our society people are beginning to prepare for that role with elderly parents who are living longer than they used to and yet need help later in life, it is not the same as having to do so suddenly after brain injury. Yet, brain injury is one of the frequent causes leading to the need for help.

You can inform them that the scenario they face is actually common. A frequent cause of traumatic brain injury is falling, particularly among older people. However, prime-of-life parents can also have a brain injury. Most children find it difficult to be the decision maker for parents who may be in the prime of life. Perhaps they are a young adult having to make financial (e.g., liquidate a family business, sell the family home, pay parents' bills) and health care (e.g., do not resuscitate, select a nursing home) decisions for a prime-of-life parent.

In such instances, sometimes there is a spouse who takes on the responsibilities for decision making, but there either may be no spouse (or partner) or they may be unable to assume this role due to emotional turmoil, inadequate skills, or lack of knowledge. In such instances, they, as adult children, can find themselves being the ultimate decision maker.

If so, remind them to take their time. Advise them to get help in figuring out what decisions are urgent and which ones can be made with more thought. Some decisions are very complex and need expert input. Emphasize that:

- They likely have no prior knowledge about brain injury, courses of recovery, and treatment/placement options. They can avoid misjudgments by learning from the experience of others conveyed through rehabilitation providers.

- They may face issues related to their parent's insurance, finances, health care directives, etc. Again their rehabilitation professionals or state Brain Injury Association can provide them with information on lawyers and financial planners who specialize in such issues after brain injury.

Third, be aware that they may have pre-onset relationship issues between them and their parent that are brought to the surface by the injury. *Reassure them that they are not alone in this regard.* Injury may raise numerous issues regarding old resentments, differences in values, lack of respect, etc. It can prove very challenging to cope simultaneously with old issues and new ones raised by the injury. However it is easier when they are honest with themselves about their old feelings and how the injury impacts them.

Sometimes they may feel that perhaps the opportunity is lost now to resolve old hurts. Alternatively, maybe they feel that this is a chance to reconnect. Regardless, they ought not to be surprised when the injury churns up their emotions. Suggest that they take this as a chance to evaluate their old perspectives and see if they still fit the new situation. This need not be done quickly, however.

Friends

Friendship after brain injury is a challenge. The person with a brain injury may think differently, act differently, and feel differently. Their friends may:

- Be unable to participate in some of the pursuits that they did together before the injury (e.g., contact sports)
- Be restricted from doing other activities (e.g., alcohol consumption)
- Have symptoms (e.g., fatigue) that may interfere with participation in activities
- Not be able to drive

- Not be able to talk or understand well

- Act in a way that embarrasses them (e.g., social inappropriateness)

Explain to them that it is common for friends to feel torn. They may experience regret at the loss of the relationship they had before the brain injury, while feeling sympathy for their friend's situation; simultaneously, they may feel unsure about how to maintain a friendship with this altered person, experiencing guilt if they decrease involvement.

Let them know that the typical pattern is early involvement with decreasing involvement as time passes: most people with brain injury lose most of their friends over the years. As their own life advances (i.e., career, marriage, children), their friend's life course may be quite different, with decreasing shared life experiences.

They are likely to want to talk with you about what to do. The following advice can help them:

- It is likely that their friend's injury will be a time of exploration for them of *their* needs, *their* values, and *their* capabilities. They can take this as a time of self-reflection, not driven by guilt or other people's expectations, but by their own desire to understand themselves. In this way, let the brain injury provide some good.

- If they can invest in long-term support of their friend with the injury, do so.

- It is all right to be intensively supportive early and to be less so as time progresses. This is common.

- It is all right to grieve for their friend and not be able to handle being involved very much. This does not make them a bad person; it makes them normal.

- It is all right to be confused. After all, usually everyone surrounding a person with brain injury is uncertain early on.

Tell them to do what they can for their friend and be honest with themselves about what they can do. There are no wrong choices.

Employers[1]

Many people lose their jobs after brain injury. This is unfortunate since so many people tie their self-worth to their job. A number of scenarios arise that you should be familiar with:

- Some persons with brain injury return to work too soon before sufficient cognitive skills return, whereas if they had waited longer, particularly during the first year after injury, for more cognitive recovery, it may have gone better.

- The employer feels that the position cannot be kept vacant long enough because of the need to have the work completed.

- The employer feels that they are unable to design accommodations that would facilitate return to work.

- The job is truly beyond the altered capabilities of the employee.

- The employer is insufficiently committed to the employee to help address the brain injury.

As employers, there are many types of relationships they might have had with the person who sustained the brain injury. These include close colleague, supervisor of a valued employee, instructor of a sub-par performer, etc. The relationship they had with their employee will likely color their own emotional responses to the brain injury. It is important for you to understand this relationship in talking with employers. *Most of the time the challenge for employers is to manage their own conflicting emotions.*

What dilemmas might you encounter? Suppose the employee is a trusted company leader now unable to perform. Do they feel an obligation to the person and, simultaneously, remorse at the corporate decision they face if the person cannot perform? Imagine the employee was a problem worker. Do they experience both relief at the person's inability to return

---

[1] All employers should be aware of the requirements of the Americans with Disabilities Act, its Amendments, and any other related laws. Nothing stated here is intended to give advice contrary to any law as it relates to persons with brain injury and the authors support adherence to all relevant laws.

to work and guilt over their feelings? Theirs is not an easy role as human beings and employers.

As with other people in the life of the person with brain injury, they face juggling compassion and reality: their emotions and competing demands. What do they feel best doing and what can they handle? There are no clear answers.

Know, however, that unlike family and friends who may attend to their expectations for themselves, discounting the limits of what they are really capable of providing long term, employers tend to focus on the "reality" of work, failing to attend to the emotional cost to themselves of the choices they make. It is the opposite scenario.

The place to start with conflicted employers, as with everyone else discussed in this book, is the opportunity to discover themselves. If they focus just on the issue of return to work, they may find themselves very emotionally distressed.

Have them be explicit about their competing drives. This will be brought out by having them complete the exercise in the companion book. If the exercise highlights conflict, have them reflect on their abilities to help and to run their business. There are no wrong decisions. Each solution *is* different. Some persons with brain injury cannot return to their old jobs; some can return with help. Some employers, just like other normal people, cannot handle brain injury; others can.

There is one final thought to bear in mind that they might not have thought about. If they are unable to have the employee return to their company, they might still be of help. After all, most employers articulate to their employees that they do not want just a "do the work — here is their paycheck" relationship. When a brain injury happens to one of their employees, it is an opportunity to demonstrate to that employee and all of their other employees what they meant, by truly following through on their idea of a broader relationship.

They might consider developing an ongoing supportive involvement with the person with a brain injury, apart from being an employer. This might help their own sense of loss and be a boon to the person with a brain injury. Imagine a person with brain injury being able to say:

"My boss couldn't take me back to work, but my boss became involved in my life, becoming a friend, emotional confidant, and advocate."

Summary

Support those with relationships to persons with brain injury by knowing that brain injury alters relationships with spouses, parents, friends, employers, etc. Moreover, as an individual in a relationship (spouse, partner, parent, friend, employer) with a person with brain injury, it will change *them*. They will be affected by the injury in ways they are likely unprepared for. It is best to be honest with them about the impact on their thoughts and feelings. They will need help to articulate their own needs and to be realistic about how they can help. Direct them to provide what help they can; care for themselves; do not feel guilty. Everyone gives to the degree they can. There are many "hidden heroes": people who work on behalf of someone with a brain injury. Suggest that they take pride in their efforts and also take care of themselves.

Lesson 8 *Getting Support*

Overview

This Lesson is intended to educate persons with brain injury about the support they can get from other people apart from the help they receive through professional counseling or family and friends. The goal is to address hurdles they may have about seeking support from other people. This Lesson will explore the types of support available and the advantages of pursuing such support. It will prepare them to seek support and explain how to go about it.

In Lesson 7 the focus was on obtaining professional help. This Lesson focuses on using other resources. There are five major ideas that you will want to convey:

1. Support groups can be very helpful in responding to brain injury.

2. Support groups offer different help than do families and friends, and both are important.

3. Family and friends may not be able to provide as much support as they need.

4. They can prepare for support groups so that they have a valuable experience.

5. Their family may want to go to their own support group.

Rationale

1. Many persons with brain injury struggle to respond to brain injury even with professional help.

2. Families and friends sometimes cannot answer the questions that persons with brain injury have. They may also have their own issues or be geographically distant. Age differences may interfere with communication between persons with brain injury and family members. There may be pre-existing conflicts that interfere with family closeness, and there may be issues with close friends if they were involved in the onset of brain injury.

3. Support groups offer a nonthreatening environment for passive observation and learning or active self-disclosure.

4. Attending support groups, particularly the first time, requires confidence that many persons with brain injury lack.

5. Teaching persons with brain injury about support groups and preparing them can decrease the emotional barriers to participation.

Presenting the Goals of This Lesson

Some persons with brain injury may not even want to discuss support groups, have preconceived ideas, or even have already had bad experiences with support groups. Hence, in presenting the goals for this Lesson, you should explain that it is worth the time to explore support groups so that they do not deprive themselves of an opportunity to ease their response to disability. Let them know that whatever concerns they might have are common, and you can explore those feelings together.

Review the following goals of the Lesson with persons with brain injury:

- To explore shortcomings they may have in their support network
- To learn what a support group can provide them
- To understand what to look for in a support group
- To prepare for going to a support group
- To know what other options they have

Repeat that it is worth the effort to fully appreciate support groups.

Addressing Common Responses to Support Groups

Below are some common responses to the idea of support groups. You can help persons with brain injury by relating that many persons with brain injury are initially hesitant to consider a support group but that, if they find the right group, the experience of the support group can be fulfilling. If the persons with brain injury are reluctant to consider a support group, ask if any of these sentiments match their feelings.

"I don't want to hear about other people's problems."

"I am uncomfortable telling other people about me."

"No one at the meeting will be like me."

"All they will want to do there is complain."

"Guest speakers usually do not address my situation."

Most people who contemplate going to a support group express sentiments similar to those above. This should not be surprising because going to a support group is a further leap into the unknown of coping with a brain injury. Yet, support groups can be a tremendously powerful tool for recovery, both for them and their family (or friends).

The power of using support group resources can be seen in some typical statements from support group participants. Contrast for the persons with brain injury the following feelings with those documented above:

"I realize that my problems are familiar to other people at my group. It makes me feel less odd."

"I am so at ease talking with people at my group. They understand me."

"I have learned that we all share similar experiences."

"In my group, if someone has a complaint or problem, we give them the opportunity to gain perspective and generate solutions."

"I like that my group chooses guest speakers together so that all of our members can hear speakers that address their needs."

Help them see that those who attend support groups have found that the feelings at the start of this Lesson often prove to be false. Encourage them that this Lesson will help them find a support group that will make them believe in their benefit.

Explaining Support Groups

Introduce this material by explaining that support groups exist for lots of different purposes. These reasons include emotional support, social activity, education, referral information, etc. Some groups may meet multiple needs.

Instruct them that they may find themselves uncertain as to exactly what needs they want to meet by attending a group until they start going. Then they may decide that a different style of group than the one they first choose is better for them. For many people, and groups, focusing on education and social activity is less threatening than addressing emotional needs, but directly discussing emotions can be the most important service of a group. Educate them to be careful to avoid selecting a group that allows them to hide from the therapeutic benefits of emotional exploration by only pursuing other activities.

It is likely to be beneficial to write down what needs they have that a support group might meet. Have them do so using the exercise in the companion book.

In an ideal world, their pre-existing support network of friends and family could meet all of their needs. Yet, many people who experience brain injury find that this is not so. Their support network may be under considerable stress itself as its members adjust to their injury. Also, their family members may focus on immediate needs such as physical care, transportation, financial resources, etc., and be too overwhelmed to additionally attend to their emotional needs. Let them know that it is all right if their family and friends struggle to meet their emotional needs. That is what support groups can help with.

Let them know that it is easy to feel let down if as time progresses they see friends moving on with their own lives and being less available to them. Furthermore, family and friends, who are unlikely to be familiar with brain injury before their injury, probably lack the knowledge to offer them education and referral information. This is common, so establishing additional relationships can be of assistance.

Even when people are available to support them emotionally, their suggestions can sometimes be unhelpful. Comments such as "You should feel lucky to be alive" or "If you try harder you can do it" can be counterproductive since such comments invalidate the struggles they may be facing. Reassurance from you that they may want to discount these perspectives can help.

You may need to explore with them why these statements are so troublesome. The idea that "you have to accept this" may be frustrating in that (1) it fails to tell them *how* to reach acceptance, and (2) implies that acceptance after brain injury is easy to achieve. Finally, many people they know may have their *own* need for them to be okay and that may influence the ability of these people to support them when they are not okay (i.e., if persons with brain injury are struggling, it may cause guilt or helpless feelings for others who need the persons with brain injury to do well, so they can feel okay themselves).

If the persons with brain injury feel that perhaps there is something out there that could help in ways different from their current support network, maybe their current support system has fallen victim to common shortcomings such networks experience. To see if this is so, have them complete the exercise in the companion book.

People have a need to see other people overcome life obstacles. This may stem from their own insecurities about feeling vulnerable to injury themselves. In the same fashion that no one likes to talk about death, people sometimes find that those with a disability remind them of their own mortality: we all prefer to live comfortably with an "invulnerability myth"—it can never happen to us! Use the term "invulnerability myth," and its destruction, to convey how much their injury may have changed the people around them.

Remind them that, of course, there are lots of truly supportive family and friends. In truth, when they are able to provide emotional nurturing and help, they are likely to prove to be their best source of encouragement. Even during the rehabilitation phase of their recovery discussed in

Lesson 3, family and friends can afford them coping support different from professionals:

- They know them more intimately and can connect with them more personally.

- They have built up trust with them over years.

Still, suggest that even if they have a wonderful network, support groups can supplement their efforts; if they do not have a network that functions well, support groups can facilitate their recovery.

Relating What They Can Gain from a Support Group

They may question what they will gain by going to a group: answer this inquiry by saying they can gain a sense of normality! Have them remember that literally millions of people have brain injuries. Theirs is a common condition. The fact that so far they may have met people who know little about brain injury does not alter the truth that so many people either have had brain injuries or are family members, friends, neighbors, co-workers, etc., of persons with brain injury. They are not alone, despite feeling that way sometimes, and a support group can help them realize that. Review the following functions of support groups to assist them to see their value:

- A support group can serve as a place where they need not feel defensive about their injury or its impact (e.g., being forgetful, not working, getting divorced). At their group they will not have to cover up problems; they can relax, be themselves, and feel all right. Support groups allow them to dispel guilt and anxiety.

- Support groups afford them the opportunity to obtain feedback. Since the other support group attendees are not otherwise in their life, they can receive unbiased feelings about their ideas and plans. Honesty is invaluable and hard to find.

- Because the members of the support group share their brain injury experience, they will want them to do well. Support group members care about each other.

- As they continue in their group they will discover that they, too, can offer guidance and help to other people, something that will make them feel good about themselves!

Instructing on What Topics Support Groups Address

Support groups address numerous issues. It is impossible to list them all. Show them Box 8.1 in the companion book that provides examples of reoccurring topics that people often seek help for from support groups. Have them put a check next to the topics they want a group to address. There are spaces at the bottom of the list to add concerns that they might want to raise for discussion at a support group meeting. Indicate that if they have an additional concern that is not already on the list, then other people in their group probably have a similar concern and will appreciate their bringing up the topic.

They can also just check off topics as their group discusses them. Doing so may help them recall the discussions when they are outside of their group.

Discussing What Support Groups Are Not

Make sure that they keep in mind that support groups are not a replacement for professional help. There are times when serious issues of adjustment arise (depression, fear/anxiety, mistrust/paranoia, suicidal/self-injurious ideation or behavior, significant guilt and anger, loss of self-esteem, marital discord, aggression, etc.) that require professional insight, knowledge, and resources. Still, support groups can be a wonderful adjunct to counseling or, for many, a sufficient means of support.

You should talk with them about support groups being an inappropriate place for romance. They should avoid going to a group with plans to make dating contacts. Group members want to feel secure and safe. The group is a support group, not a singles club. They may make other people uncomfortable if they solicit them.

On the other hand, inform them that, of course, friendships do develop out of support groups. That is one of their benefits. However, dating and romance introduce complications. Provide them with the insight that if their relationship goes badly they risk losing their support group, too, because it can become awkward to attend if their ex-dating partner is there. Even if their relationship goes well, and they both continue to participate in the same group, their relationship will change how they act and what they say during the group.

Teach them to not take their support group resource lightly by assuming that it would be easy to replace. Their support group members are an important resource for them: have them be careful not to squander that resource.

Instructing Them What to Look for in a Support Group

Telling them what they will find most satisfying in a support group would presuppose that everyone's needs are the same. Actually, the diversity of needs is as broad as the circumstances and effects of brain injury. In addition, their needs may change over time. Nevertheless, there are variables that they can consider when selecting a support group. Each person can individually decide how to rate each support group on each variable.

Let them know you will review with them variables to consider when selecting a support group.

Type of Members

Tell them that there are two types of groups:

- Persons with brain injury only (often called a "peer support group")
- Mixed groups that also include family members

Summarize for them that the primary advantage of a peer support group is that it provides them the opportunity to have unvarnished discussions.

- They can discuss issues that they may have *about* their family or concerns they may have *for* their family.
- They may be angry or disappointed with their family and they may want a place where they can vent those feelings.
- They may be worried about their family members and how they are doing.
- A group without family members can provide them with an avenue to express their fears safely.

There are also advantages to a mixed group.

- They can hear how other families are handling issues.
- They may learn that their family issues are very common.
- Their family, if they attend with them, may see how other persons with brain injury and their families function, giving them a new perspective on their interactions with the persons with brain injury.
- Their family may hear concerns raised by other people, but important to them, without the persons with brain injury having to introduce the topic. This can open the door for them to have a discussion with their family. The group discussion can give them and their family a common jumping off point for future private talks (e.g., "Remember what was said at the meeting last week by Sally? I feel the same way sometimes.").

Advise them that they need not choose between these two groups. They could attend one of each for different needs. (Make them aware that their family may want to also attend a family-only group without them. It is best to avoid being hurt by this. Recommend that they recognize that families have needs, too, and may want privacy to care for themselves.)

Group Facilitator Qualities

Once they select the type of group, they need to consider the group facilitator. Support groups can be run by a:

- Professional
- Family member
- Person with a brain injury

Encourage them that there is no clear answer as to who is best. In part, it depends on whether the group is for families or persons with brain injury, for educational purposes or for support, for help early or late in recovery, etc. Each type of facilitator (professional, family member, or person with a brain injury) potentially brings strengths and limitations to the facilitator role. Have them reflect on who they will feel most comfortable with running their group. In each category of facilitator there are excellent facilitators, and there are those who are limited in their abilities to facilitate a group.

Next, have them determine the qualities of the support group facilitator that best appeal to them. Typically, most people want a facilitator who is experienced, knowledgeable, supportive, not too directive, but able to facilitate communication. They may find it useful to inquire about any training the facilitator has had in running a support group (e.g., instruction through their state chapter of the Brain Injury Association of America).

Most groups function best when facilitators avoid trying to obtain *their* own emotional support through the groups they facilitate. Facilitators ought to be able to serve the needs of their groups without their own needs interfering.

Box 8.2 in the companion book provides a brief checklist of facilitator characteristics to consider. It is all right to ask facilitators about their style, experience, and knowledge. Have them complete this checklist of what they want from a facilitator.

Of course, it may be difficult to fully determine all of the information in the above checklist before going to a few meetings, though they may obtain an impression of facilitators by talking with them first. Still, the list can help guide their impressions after a few meetings. It may be useful to attend different groups to see which facilitator feels most comfortable to them.

Group Structure

Explain that some groups attempt to structure meetings, whereas other groups are open-ended. Groups with structure may aim to address topics sequentially across meetings or they may structure time within a meeting (e.g., if a speaker is coming). The advantage of having structure is that the group insures it will cover important topics that otherwise might be missed.

Open-ended groups are more likely to pursue the immediate needs of its members within meetings or across meetings. Pertinent frustrations or concerns can be more quickly addressed. However, topics that are worrisome, but that no one immediately raises, may get overlooked.

Let persons with brain injury know, of course, that group structure can change over time and that some groups combine structured and unstructured time. Either group is fine; it is personal preference.

Practical Considerations

Make sure that they give thought to practical considerations when they select a group, too. Have them think about:

- The location of the group. Some groups meet at hospitals; some groups meet at religious sites. They must decide if they are comfortable in these locations.

- Whether the building the group meets in is accessible if they have mobility variables to consider.

- The time of day and day of the week; a great support group that they do not actually attend is worthless.

- Transportation needs that may be a factor.

- The duration of the meeting: too long and they may fatigue; too short and little is addressed.

- The frequency of the group: too often and it can be difficult to attend; too infrequent and it might not meet their needs.

- Donations, if any, to maintain the group (e.g., postage for mailing announcements, copying notices, refreshments).

Have them use Box 8.3 in the companion book to select factors that are important to them as they select a group.

Advising Them about How Soon They Should Go

Hopefully they received information about support groups during their initial rehabilitation. In fact, many professionals anticipate that they will want to go shortly after discharge.

- They may find that connecting with other people early is a great source of comfort and reassurance.

For some people this may be unrealistic.

- They may feel too overwhelmed following discharge to add a support group meeting to their agenda.

- They might need some time out of the hospital to see what life will be like—and what challenges they will face—and how they feel about things.

Guide them that it is okay if they do not go right away, but that their professionals will tend to be concerned that, if they fail to start soon, they will never get around to going at all or that they will forget to arrange to go. Suggest to them that if they do not start in a group shortly after hospital discharge, it is a good idea to plan a time when they will re-visit going, perhaps about six months after rehabilitation hospital discharge.

Point out that by six months they should have some idea of how they are feeling and whether their network is supplying them with all of their support needs. Then, if they choose not to start going to a support group, they should revisit this idea every six months for a few years. It would be a good idea to write down in Box 8.4 in the companion book the dates to consider a support group.

(Not everyone with a brain injury has been hospitalized. Some people are seen at emergency rooms and are released. Other people never go to an emergency room. If they are one of these people with a brain injury, they too can contemplate going to a support group. The benefits are awaiting them, also. When they choose to go depends on their personal situation and needs.)

Getting Them Prepared

They may feel some fear when they think about attending a support group. Reflecting with them ahead of time about a few key issues may relieve much of their anxiety. Remind them that everyone there has had a brain injury, and while their exact circumstance may not be precisely the same as theirs, they likely share many of the same experiences. Moreover, even if they had unique experiences, the people at the group are there, in part, to help them. Everyone came, just as they will, to learn, but also to help.

They may be worried about their ability or desire, at least initially, to disclose personal information and feelings. Ask them if they will feel uncomfortable talking in front of other people. If so, let them know that these are normal concerns. Telling them the following may help make them more comfortable:

- They are not obligated to talk or disclose information, though the group may ask them to introduce themselves. They can tell the group, particularly for the first meeting, that they are nervous and want to get more comfortable before participating a lot.

- They may discover a desire to participate earlier than they might anticipate when they observe how comfortably the group handles issues just like the ones they confront.

- As time progresses their hesitancy may decrease as they become familiar with their group members.

Still, if self-disclosure is a particular worry of theirs, suggest that they discuss it ahead of time with the group facilitator. Tell them to find out what the ground rules are: ask if everyone has to talk.

Review Why People Stop Going to a Support Group

People tend to drop out of support groups. Perhaps they can avoid this pitfall if you review with them beforehand the reasons that lead some people to stop attending so that they can be ready to sidestep those traps:

- They should avoid the illusion that a support group will immediately make them feel better. Becoming more resilient takes time and it requires real life practice of the insights they gain at meetings. In fact, personal self-disclosure, listening to others, and gaining insight can be emotionally painful. On the whole, they should find a support group to be "supportive," but there can be meetings that are emotionally trying.

- They will likely find support groups to be disappointing if they are looking for people who will feel sorry for them. They will find empathetic people, but not people who readily tolerate self-pity. Therefore, some people leave groups because they are unready to transition from despair to acceptance.

- Some people stop attending support groups because they do not want to be with other persons with brain injury. They may find it too hard to see other people with disabilities. They may learn about problems they did not know could occur. They may not be ready to admit how similar to "those people" they are. Attending a support group entails some degree of acceptance (as defined in previous Lessons). Of course, if they are struggling with denial, then a support group may be just the place for them to get help with acceptance.

- They may quit a support group because they are afraid to trust, and attending a support group involves trust. If they are going to disclose their concerns (e.g., fears, worries) and their successes, then they need to believe the support group members will treat them gently and support them.

- They may feel lonely and want just the social aspect of a group and they may find that the emotional discussions are too intense.
- They may find that there was just not a good match of personalities in a particular group.

If these reasons for leaving their group fit them, encourage them to not give up on support groups. Rather, suggest that they locate a new group where they fit better and can trust the people in the group.

Of course, logistical concerns can also turn out to influence attendance more than they thought they would:

- It can be challenging to arrange reliable transportation.
- Periodic medical flare-ups could interfere too much.
- Other life responsibilities (e.g., work) could conflict with meetings.
- They could struggle with fatigue.
- It may be too much to add in one more appointment.

Whatever their issues in this regard, it would be wise to have them contemplate how they can restructure things so as to maximize their attendance.

They may also discontinue attendance because they obtained what they needed from the group.

- They received the information they needed to resolve particular issues.
- They came to sufficient terms with their injury for now.
- They re-established a personal support network that meets their needs.

Of course, some of the people who leave groups periodically return when life circumstances change. Remind them that they can always resume attending. Alternatively, they may leave their support group to join other ones because they need a different type of group providing a different experience; maybe they are at different points in their lives now than when they started in their groups. Finally, some people discontinue going to a support group to start their own group as a facilitator.

Whatever their reasons are for leaving a group, counsel them that they should avoid feeling guilty about doing so. It *is* difficult to succeed in life with a brain injury. Whether their reasons for stopping are logistical or interpersonal, have them give themselves credit for doing the best they can. Life after brain injury is an experiment: they need to figure out what works best for them. Perhaps a different group would be better for them or a group sometime in the future (or maybe support groups are just not for them). Regardless, make sure they make an informed decision and are satisfied with their choice.

Introducing the Individual Peer Support Option

They may find that a group environment is not for them, but that they would like to talk with someone else with a brain injury. Instruct them that what they may be looking for is a "peer mentor." A peer mentor is someone they establish a relationship with beyond just being friends. It is like having someone to talk with who has more experience with brain injury than they have and has reached a level of comfort and coping with brain injury. Relate to them that whereas professional counselors can impart wisdom to them from having seen what worked for many other people with brain injury, peer mentors impart insight from their personal experiences. If peer mentors have been successful in coping, then peer mentors can serve as role models for them.

Remind them that they should use the same care in selecting a peer mentor as they would when screening a support group facilitator. Direct persons with brain injury to consider the variables in Box 8.5 in the companion book.

Tell them that it is best if they arrange for a peer mentor through an organization so that they have some assurance that the mentor is reputable and has their best interest at heart. They want someone who (1) has been trained as a mentor and (2) is emotionally doing well.

They can start by making inquiries at their local hospital or their state Brain Injury Association.

Finally, educate them that a peer mentor, a professional counselor, and a support group are different resources for them. They are not mutually exclusive—they can have all or any combination as resources at any time.

Linking Them with the Brain Injury Association

Regardless of whether they attend a support group, it is wise for you to advise them to join their state Brain Injury Association. These chapters of the non-profit Brain Injury Association of America can provide support, networking, advocacy, referral, and information. Have them ask to be placed on their state Brain Injury Association and Brain Injury Association of America mailing lists for newsletters and announcements. They will probably be amazed at the assistance and support the people at the state Brain Injury Association can provide them.

Warning Them about the Internet

Some people seek support over the internet in online chat rooms or groups. Caution them to be extremely careful about online support activities. They must protect themselves. After all, they are seeking support at a time when they may be emotionally vulnerable and it is easy for someone to take advantage of them. They can be emotionally harmed by anonymous people who have hidden motives. Some people on the internet may also try to financially abuse them, and if they ever arrange to meet in person, they can be hurt physically.

Advise them that it is probably best to attend support groups that are real, not virtual, and that are recommended by recognized organizations (e.g., their local hospital or their state Brain Injury Association). However, sometimes a recognized organization may run a support group over the phone by conference call. Make sure that the organization is reputable (i.e., check with their local hospital or their state Brain Injury Association).

You can advise them that there is however some excellent information about brain injury available over the internet. Still, they must be cautious about what they believe. Again caution them that *anyone* can put information online. A fancy website with great graphics and an official sounding name does not mean the information is accurate. Some people online have an axe to grind or just do not know what they are talking about.

Nevertheless, the internet is valuable. First, it can help them generate questions to ask their professionals or it can raise issues that they can bring to their support group. Second, there are some sites that they can feel more secure in trusting. Good places to start would be their state Brain Injury Association website or the Brain Injury Association of America website (as of this writing, www.biausa.org).

Addressing the Family Needs for a Support Group

There is one last thought for you to raise: even if they choose to defer attending a support group, their family members may feel that it is helpful for *the family members* to go to a group. This varies from family to family. Review with them the following: it may help their family when the family members:

- Feel scared and need reassurance
- Are angry and need support
- Need to take a little time to care for themselves
- Need validation of their decision making

Of course, just like persons with brain injury, their family may want to wait awhile:

- They may be juggling work, child rearing, visits to the hospital, meeting with lawyers, etc.
- It may be too overwhelming to add a support group.

Finally, you should make them aware that it may be difficult for their family members to go to a support group, even one just for families.

- The idea of a support group may challenge the family members' sense of competency. They may find it hard to admit their own neediness. Going to a group may heighten their own sense of vulnerability. They may be afraid that they will fall apart emotionally, after learning to be strong for the persons with brain injury, once they are in an environment where it is all right to admit to their own feelings.

- Guilt can be a big factor that reduces support group attendance by family members. Some family members may feel guilty about spending time caring for themselves, believing that they should focus all of their energy on the persons with brain injury. Such family members typically have adopted the role of "nurturer" (see Lesson 7) after their loved one's injury. However, without support they risk burnout.

- Other family members feel guilty about not having been able to protect the persons with brain injury from harm in life and support group attendance would entail confronting their feeling of having failed. Such family members often have adopted the role of "breadwinner" (see Lesson 7) after their injury. They may compensate for their perceived failure by working at their jobs to gain more money for the persons with brain injury. They may try to marshal resources to be better able to shield the persons with brain injury from the impact to their life of their injury and from harm in the future. However, they risk feeling inadequate without support.

- If family members were angry with the persons with brain injury over their pre-onset lifestyle or other factors, they may feel remorse about not having had a better relationship with them before their brain injury. Perhaps they now regret their anger, or even their disappointment, and cannot face their own shortcomings in their relationship with the person with brain injury. They may fear that a support group will bring forth their regrets (maybe in tearful self-disclosure). Such family members risk depression without support.

- Apart from guilt, some family members may have feelings of tremendous loss themselves. Family members who were proud of the person with brain injury and had invested in this person's accomplishments may actually experience a blow to their own ego and esteem. Moreover, if they participated a great deal in the person's life, the gap left in their own lives can be a source of uncertainty for them about how to live now. These family members may be embarrassed to disclose such feelings; it is difficult to admit how much of their happiness and satisfaction depended on this person who has changed so much. However, these family members risk feeling empty without support.

Inquire if it is surprising to think about issues of guilt, loss, and coping by their family. The preceding paragraphs may even have made them feel guilty. There is good news. First, their family members are responsible for their own feelings: the persons with brain injury are not. Second, what is done is done: they cannot fix the past, but they can work together to have a better future together. Third, there is help available to their family. The persons with brain injury can encourage their family to attend a support group for themselves!

Summary

Regardless of how they get support (personal network, support group, peer mentor, professional counseling, etc.) you can remind them that they are not alone. Brain injury happens to huge numbers of people every year. However, it gets little newspaper space or television time and what is conveyed by the press is often misleading. It is easy for them to come to believe that literally no one else has had any of their experiences or could understand their worries. Encourage the idea that there are lots of people ready to help them.

Lesson 9   *How to Keep on Recovering Well*

Overview

There are three focuses for the therapist in this Lesson. First, you will be helping readers with brain injury integrate all they have learned and discovered through reading the companion book and participating in the process of self-discovery through its multiple exercises. With your guidance this Lesson should help clients combine their new awareness of their unique pattern of post-injury strengths and deficits with facts and skills they have learned related to recovering from and living with brain injury. Clients with brain injury who are able to accomplish this combined application will go forward as more discriminating and aware consumers who can seek, select, and apply the specific strategies and supports that they need. A second focus is helping clients with brain injury develop a personal plan for maintaining and strategically using their injury-related knowledge and the multiple strategies and coping methods demonstrated and recommended. Third, you should work to bolster clients' ability to sustain a positive inner voice and outlook.

Rationale

1. Clients may receive comprehensive inpatient rehabilitation after brain injury, but many are discharged quickly, still having moderate to severe neurobehavioral and cognitive deficits.

2. The health care literature tells us that clients with a variety of diseases and disabilities find support groups helpful and comforting. Providing clients with brain injury with links to the larger community of persons living with brain injury will increase their available resources and supports.

3. Clients with brain injury have special learning needs and repetition of helpful concepts and guidance increases their potential for coping and adjustment.

4. Clients with brain injury often encounter fragmented outpatient rehabilitation services or have limited insurance coverage for outpatient services. They have continuing needs for information and coping strategies because these will not be as consistently available to them after inpatient discharge.

5. Clients with brain injury have impaired attention, memory, and problem-solving abilities. After completing rehabilitation, they benefit from supports for sustaining their consistent use of compensatory and coping strategies.

6. Clients with brain injury often achieve maximal benefit of rehabilitation after 18 months to 2 years. After this time, their need for supports for living in the community often remain or intensify.

Presenting the Goals of This Lesson

Review the following goals with the client.

- Help clients describe their personal profile of post-injury strengths and weaknesses

- Identify which of the many strategies learned will help each individual challenge

- Consistently keep a positive inner voice during the challenges now and in the future

- Describe the network of persons and resources available in the community and nation as recovery continues

Recovering Well!

Readers with brain injury who have gotten this far in their books may now wonder whether we will tell them that their challenges are over. You will have to explain that no, for most people with brain injury, the challenges continue. However, you can reassure them that reading the companion book and completing the exercises has led to increased awareness and understanding that will help their continued recovery. In particular, tell clients that Lesson 9 will help them review, integrate, and apply all that they have learned so far. Explain that Lesson 9 will also introduce and present the combined wisdom of many persons in the wider community of consumers, some of whom have been living with brain injury for many years. This wider community of surviving persons with brain injury has shared their experiences, best advice, and insider knowledge about living successfully with brain injury and the pitfalls to avoid. Also mention that Lesson 9 will help them develop doable plans to implement all of the ideas they have practiced in the preceding Lessons. Your primary recommendation for clients will be to consistently use the life-long healthy coping habits described in Lessons 1 to 8. This guiding principle will be carefully detailed using two sources. Explain to clients that you will not only review what providers and brain injury researchers have learned about living well after brain injury, but will also tell them what people with brain injury recommend. Broad, general strategies and ideas for proactive solutions to common problems will be described and demonstrated. You will be assisting clients with developing doable plans for living life successfully after brain injury.

Reviewing What Has Been Learned

Remind clients that they have covered lots of topics as they read through and participated in the suggested exercises of Lessons 1 to 8. Show them the titles and content highlights of all earlier Lessons using Box 9.1, Lesson 9, of the companion book. Therapists can use Box 9.1 in Lesson 9 as a shorthand framework for reviewing major concepts and strategies within each of the past Lessons. It will be important to relate the review to clients' unique needs and issues as you have come to know them. Ask them if they have any questions and if they have understood the content of each Lesson, both while they were originally reading it and now, while you are reviewing it. If the therapist believes that clients have not fully grasped or do not remember the content or how to use the strategies suggested, they should make an effort to re-explain or demonstrate any of these again. Use the companion book to go back over these multiple concepts and strategies they have learned through their reading and their participation in the book's exercises. Build links for clients between the unique challenges and questions they have uncovered in their sessions and the information and ideas in the book. Your care in establishing these links will increase the likelihood that clients will understand that the strategies can help and that the book can be an ongoing resource for them. Reviewing the concepts and ideas in the order of the Lessons will be best for providing a structure and model for clients to follow on their own.

Listening to the Voices of the Wider Brain Injury Community

No book about recovering from brain injury would be complete without telling persons with brain injury about the experiences of other people in the community who have been living with it, sometimes for many years. Explain that when persons living with brain injury talk to professionals and others, their comments fall into two major categories: their pet peeves and their best advice for living. Explain that Lesson 9 will present both what community-dwelling persons with brain injury have told others about their biggest annoyances and challenges, and their best advice for living with brain injury. Tell clients that you will first learn how people living with brain injury deal with day-to-day frustrations in the community. Direct clients to Box 9.2, Lesson 9, in their books entitled "Survivors of Brain Injury Tell Us …." Talk about how there is a positive spin for every pet peeve. Emphasize that community-dwelling persons with brain injury recommend countering these negatives with strong positives and counting their blessings.

Developing a Plan to Continue the Journey of Recovering Well Day to Day

Tell clients that ongoing steps to progress and adjustment will involve developing a personal, doable plan for continuing to improve and rejoin the community in a satisfying, productive manner. State that their work with their book has helped them identify their own unique pattern of post-injury cognitive and behavioral assets and challenges. Explain that the best way for them to continue to get better is to use what they have learned in combination with using a proactive rather than a reactive approach. If they are proactive, they will plan ahead and think in action words. If they react, it will be after the fact and usually not as productive. Direct their attention to Box 9.3 of Lesson 9 in their books, showing them that it contains words that will lead them toward productive daily routines and accomplishments.

Explain to client that, unlike the words "avoid," or "withdraw," the words in Box 9.3 will lead to doing something productive when consciously added to their daily vocabulary.

Direct them to *use* the headings and list in Box 9.4 for proactively ***planning*** to address any obstacles and problems they encounter now or in their future.

Recommend ***preparation*** by using any of the prior questionnaires found in Lessons 1 to 8 for helping to identify post-injury problem areas. Show clients how the list includes the headings ***Problem, Proactive Problem Solving.*** Explain that they can *use* the list to first find their problem, then follow the heading to find the suggested solutions, and finally ***develop and choose*** their own unique solution. Point out that the instructions you just gave them contained several of the boldfaced action words. Provide an example of proactive problem solving by reviewing ***Jim's Story***. Help clients study the content of Box 9.4 and think through a solution for Jim.

Jim's Story

Jim needs to start outpatient physical therapy as he is having difficulty with balance again, even though he finished his brain injury rehabilitation three months ago. His home is too far from the physical therapy center for him to get there by foot, and it would be too expensive to take a cab back and forth. He gets confused, because of his brain injury, when he tries to tell people how to get him there and then get him back home. Using Box 9.4, Lesson 9, of the companion book, under the problem "transportation," notice the solution for Jim would be to find out how to get a ride with a bus service, or a Care Van-type service.

Returning to Work or Productive Activity: Are You Ready?

Therapists should tell clients that people with brain injury want to be productive and many want to return to work. The client should be told that only about 39% of persons with TBI actually return to full time competitive employment. The reasons for this have to do with some of the cognitive and behavioral problems caused by the injury itself. Memory, extreme fatigue, impulsiveness, and concentration are among the typical problems that make it challenging for persons with brain injury to look for, find, and keep a job. Explain that persons with brain injury should ask themselves some very important questions before attempting to return to work.

1. Am I ready to work?

2. Can I afford to work?

3. Do I receive disability income that might be reduced if I work?

Tell clients that all of these questions must receive careful thought prior to looking for a job. For example, with regard to item 1, clients must be able to get to the location of work by driving or by public transportation. Endurance is another readiness consideration. Ask clients about their normal waking and sleeping hours. Ask them what time of day they feel sleepy and for how long? With regard to question 2, being able to afford going to work, tell clients that such considerations as expenses due to daycare for children, uniforms, transportation, and equipment must always be factored into a decision about working. Finally, related to item 3, explain that the choice to work is affected by disability income and the need not to jeopardize its continuation through working too many hours, which is always something to consider.

Therapists should also let clients know that there are various points along the journey back to work after brain injury, each with its own set of considerations and challenges. There is a time of just getting ready to go out there and look which involves facing any potential obstacles to working and how to overcome these if they exist. Then there is a time of actually seeking a position. Finally, once hired or once a volunteer position has started, there are special issues related to keeping that position. Therapists can help clients link with community-based agencies, clubhouses, or day programs that are specifically focused on vocational services and supports for persons with brain injury. Prepare in advance by searching for the best web addresses, information and contact numbers, and locations of these potential resources so that you can provide those to clients as part of this session. In addition, most of those organizations will have information about supported employment, which is an evidence-based help for job acquisition and stability.

Returning to Work: Obstacles and Aids to Preparing to Work

Explain to clients that when they begin to consider returning to work or starting to do volunteer work, they should try to do as much as possible to remove potential obstacles and take advantage of proactive aids to realizing their goals. Potential ***obstacles*** include sleeping late and staying up too late, not having set habits and routines, difficulty with fatigue, cognitive deficits, costs of work, and lack of confidence. Direct clients back to Lessons related to improving endurance, compensatory cognitive strategies, and proactive problem-solving for guidance in overcoming those obstacles. In addition, share with clients that aiming for regular bed times, improved sleep hygiene, better nutrition and better self-pacing will help them overcome these obstacles. Therapists should also promote avoidance of negative self-talk and setting of realistic goals. Again help clients find those prior Lessons in their books with guidance about these issues. Explore possible costs of working with clients, including daycare, uniforms, and transportation. Tell clients about potential ***aids to overcoming the obstacles*** including setting doable goals, organizing themselves, consistent and purposeful use of compensatory cognitive strategies, and use of a work mentor. With regard to the mentor, tell clients that they should look for someone who they trust, who is working, and who will give them encouraging feedback and information without asking to be paid.

Returning to Work: Actual Job Search and Application

Explain that making a good impression through first contacts, interviews, and résumés that are focused but impressive to potential employers can be challenging after brain injury. Tell clients that there are fortunately some excellent ways to improve the likelihood that they can make the best impression possible, despite difficulties with speech, memory, concentration, and nervousness. For example, explain that knowing what their strengths and weaknesses are will be critical for making sure they make a good match between their abilities, preferences, and any position they accept or seek. Guide clients back to the many questionnaires related to their specific post-injury challenges that they have taken during their reading of their books. Show them how to make a list of their strengths and their weaker areas. Following these two lists, suggest that they complete the "Vocational Decision-Making Process Form" in Box 9.5, Lesson 9, whenever they are considering a job or volunteer opportunity. Show clients how to fill out the form, first with their strengths and weaknesses, then what kind of work they like. Next ask clients if they have considered doing any particular work lately. If they are not able to name a recent job search, use a possible job like stock clerk in a drug store as a sample for demonstrating the use of the form. As an example, direct clients to Joe's Story in their book. Tell clients that stock clerks often have late afternoon or evening hours, work inside, have to record small numbers from bottles and products on to a sheet, keep track of items on aisles and replace them when they get low, etc. Ask clients to list these under the heading "My Potential Job Facts." When they finish filling in that row, ask them to compare their answers with their work preferences and strengths, and decide if the job of stock clerk would be a good match for their work preferences, skills, and weaker areas.

In terms of communication skills for work settings, guide clients back to the Lessons describing active listening techniques and best social behavior for making friends. Remind clients to improve their social relationships with active listening, making sure they do not dominate the conversation or interrupt, and with not coming on too strong. Point out that improved communication and social behavior will improve all social relationships, not just work-related relationships.

Therapists should suggest a work mentor, preferably someone who is working, who can be trusted to advise the client without asking for money, in a responsible, positive manner. Mentors can help with applications, and can look over and assist clients in developing a résumé that presents qualifications and abilities rather than leading with dates worked. Examples of these alternate formats are featured in Boxes 9.6 and 9.7 of Lesson 9.

Assist clients in trying these formats out. Help them arrange their work skills in the format to help them see how the dates become somewhat less prominent and the qualifications are highlighted. Tell them that use of these different formats will help minimize attention to work history gaps that may have occurred following the brain injury. The alternate formats will also help present the clients' abilities and qualifications in the best light possible.

Finally, for the interview itself, help clients integrate advice for social communication provided in prior Lessons. In addition, advise clients to be on time, make good eye contact, dress neatly, avoid falling asleep, avoid making inappropriate comments, and wait before answering to make sure that they have fully understood the question. Tell clients that interviews are nerve wracking for most people. People who prepare with good questions and a positive outlook will be able to manage this nervousness once they are actually in the interview. Guide clients to look back at Lessons that address stress management techniques.

Returning to Work: Enhancing Job Stability

Therapists should explain to clients that once they have a job or start volunteering there will be issues that arise that may lead to worry about keeping a job because of having a brain injury. There are stressful situations and difficult people to deal with at any job. There are demands that could lead to fatigue and a feeling of being overwhelmed. Those two statements are true for anyone, and a brain injury increases the chances that they will threaten job stability.

Tell clients that several Lessons of their book can be applied to the work setting and the day-to-day coping that is required for staying in a job. Make sure to point out that Lessons dealing with mood, coping, self-management of feelings, and problem solving hold important ideas for insuring job stability. Direct them to Box 9.1 in this Lesson. For example, tell them that relaxation techniques, positive self-talk, and taking care of oneself are strategies that make it more likely that a person with a brain injury can deal effectively with day-to-day stressors at work.

The therapist should suggest several other approaches for improving the chances of keeping a job. Tell clients that when starting a job, they should take their time to get to know the people and systems as each setting has its own way of doing things. In that way they will not run the risk of being seen as pushy and overbearing. In addition, maintaining the same good grooming, outlook, self-care, and plan for avoiding mistakes will be as important for their job stability as it was for the interview phase. Mistakes and social blunders, falling asleep on the job, and taking a haphazard approach to assigned tasks can also be avoided through careful, proactive, and consistent use of compensatory strategies covered in several of the Lessons. Therapists should assist clients in finding these specific strategies in the Lessons of their book.

Summary

As a final integrative effort, therapists should name the sections and guidance provided in Lesson 9, specifically pointing out the charts for reviewing preceding Lessons—the "Survivors of Brain Injury Tell Us …," "Action Words," "Proactive Problem Solving" charts, and the "Vocational Decision-Making Process Form"—and the purpose and potential uses for each. Congratulate clients for their work and learning through the process of reading the book and engaging in the exercises. Note that they now are armed with general wisdom about brain injury and their own unique injury and recovery story that will serve them well in their ongoing journey.

References

Lesson 1

Caplan, B., & Moelter, S. (2009). Stroke. In R. G. Frank, M. Rosenthal, B. Caplan (Eds.), *Handbook of Rehabilitation Psychology*. Washington, DC: American Psychological Association Press, pp. 75–108.

Conder, R., Evans, D., Faulkner, P., et al. (1988). An interdisciplinary programme for cognitive rehabilitation. *Brain Injury, 2*, 365–385.

Crimmons, C. (2000). *Where Is the Mango Princess? A Journey Back from Brain Injury*. New York: Random House.

Gordon, W. A., Zafonte, R., Cicerone, K., Cantor, J., Brown, M., Lombard, L. et al. (2006). Traumatic brain injury rehabilitation: State of the science. *American Journal of Physical Medicine & Rehabilitation, 85*, 343–382.

Niemeier, J. P., & Kreutzer, J. S. (2001). *First Steps Toward Recovery From Brain Injury*. Richmond, VA: National Resource Center for Traumatic Brain Injury.

Osborn, C. L. (2000). *Over My Head: A Doctor's Own Story of Head Injury from the Inside Looking Out*. Kansas City, MO: Andrews McNeel.

Patterson, D. R., & Ford, G. R. (2009). Brain injuries. In R. G. Frank, M. Rosenthal, & B. Caplan (Eds.), *Handbook of Rehabilitation Psychology*. Washington, DC: American Psychological Association Press, pp. 145–162.

Ragnarsson, K. T. (2006). Traumatic brain injury research since the 1998 NIH Consensus Conference: Accomplishments and unmet goals. *Journal of Head Trauma Rehabilitation, 21*, 379–387.

Rosenthal, M., & Ricker, J. H. (2009). Traumatic brain injury. In R. G. Frank, M. Rosenthal, & B. Caplan (Eds.), *Handbook of Rehabilitation Psychology*. Washington, DC: American Psychological Association Press, pp. 49–74.

Swanson, K. L. (2003). *I'll Carry the Fork! Recovering a Life After Brain Injury*. Scotts Valley, CA: Rising Star Press.

Taylor, J. B. (2006). *Stroke of Insight*. New York: Viking.

Willer, B., Rosenthal, M., Kreutzer, J. S., Gordon, W. A., & Rempel, R. (1993). Assessment of community integration following traumatic brain injury. *Journal of Head Trauma Rehabilitation, 8*. 75–87.

Woodruff, L. (2008). *In an Instant: A Family's Journey of Love and Healing*. New York: Random House.

Lesson 2

Cicerone, K. D., Dahlberg, C., Kalmar, K., et al. (2000). Evidence-based cognitive rehabilitation: Recommendations for clinical practice. *Archives of Physical Medicine and Rehabilitation, 81*, 1596–1615.

Cicerone, K. D., Dahlberg, C., Malec, J. F., Langenbahn, D. M., Felicetti, T., K. T., Kneipp, S., et al. (2005). Evidence-based cognitive rehabilitation: Updated review of the literature from 1998 through 2002. *Archives of Physical Medicine and Rehabilitation, 86*, 1681–1687.

Gordon, W. A., Zafonte, R., Cicerone, K., Cantor, J., Brown, M., Lombard, L. et al. (2006). Traumatic brain injury rehabilitation: State of the science. *American Journal of Physical Medicine & Rehabilitation, 85*, 343–382.

Levin, H. S., High, W. M., Goethe, K. E., Sisson, R. A., Overall, J. E., Rhoades, H. M., Eisenberg, H. M., Kalisky, Z., & Gary, H. E. (1987). The neurobehavioural rating scale: Assessment of the behavioural sequelae of head injury by the clinician. *Journal of Neurology, Neurosurgery, and Psychiatry, 50*, 183–193.

Lezak, M. D., Howieson, D. B., Loring, D. W., Hannay, H. J., & Fischer, J. S. (1995). *Neuropsychological Assessment* (3rd Ed.). New York: Oxford University Press.

Niemeier, J. P. (2002). Visual imagery training for patients with visual perceptual deficits following right hemisphere cerebrovascular accidents: A case study presenting the Lighthouse Strategy. *Rehabilitation Psychology, 47*, 426–437.

Niemeier, J. P., & Kreutzer, J. S. (2001). *First Steps Toward Recovery from Brain Injury*. Richmond, VA: National Resource Center for Traumatic Brain Injury.

Niemeier, J. P., & Burnett, D. M. (2001). No such thing as "uncomplicated bereavement" for patients in rehabilitation. *Disability and Rehabilitation, 23*, 645–653.

Niemeier, J. P., Kreutzer, J. S., & Taylor, L. A. (2005). Acute cognitive and neurobehavioral intervention for individuals with acquired brain injury: Preliminary outcome data. *Neuropsychological Rehabilitation, 15,* 129–146.

Patterson, D. R. & Ford, G. R. (2009). Brain injuries. In R. G. Frank, M. Rosenthal, & B. Caplan (Eds.), *Handbook of Rehabilitation Psychology*. Washington, DC: American Psychological Association Press, pp. 145–162.

Ragnarsson, K. T. (2006). Traumatic brain injury research since the 1998 NIH Consensus Conference: Accomplishments and unmet goals. *Journal of Head Trauma Rehabilitation, 21,* 379–387.

Raskin, S. A., & Mateer, C. A. (2000). *Neuropsychological Management of Mild Traumatic Brain Injury*. New York: Oxford University Press.

Rosenthal, M., Griffith, E. R., Kreutzer, J. S., Miller, J. D., & Bond, M. R. (Eds.) (1999). *Rehabilitation of the Adult and Child with Traumatic Brain Injury*. Philadelphia, PA: F. A. Davis.

Rosenthal, M., & Ricker, J. H. (2009). Traumatic brain injury. In R. G. Frank, M. Rosenthal, & B. Caplan (Eds.), *Handbook of Rehabilitation Psychology*. Washington, DC: American Psychological Association Press, pp. 49–74.

Ruttan, L., Martin, K., Liu, A., Colella, B., & Green, R. E. (2008). Long-term cognitive outcome in moderate to severe traumatic brain injury: A meta-analysis examining timed and untimed tests at 1 and 4.5 or more years after injury. *Archives of Physical Medicine and Rehabilitation, 89,* S69–S76.

Sohlberg, M. M., & Mateer, C. A. (2001). *Cognitive Rehabilitation: An Integrative Neuropsychological Approach*. New York: Guilford Press.

Stuss, D. T., Winocur, G., & Robertson, I. H. (1999). *Cognitive Neurorehabilitation*. New York: Cambridge University Press.

West, D., & Niemeier, J. P. (2005). *Memory Matters: Strategies for Managing Everyday Memory Problems*. Richmond, VA: National Resource Center for Traumatic Brain Injury.

Lesson 3

Brain Injury Association of America. (2007). *The Essential Brain Injury Guide* (4th Ed.). McLean, VA: Author.

Caplan, B., & Moelter, S. (2009). Stroke. In R. G. Frank, M. Rosenthal, & B. Caplan (Eds.), *Handbook of Rehabilitation Psychology*. Washington, DC: American Psychological Association Press, pp. 75–108.

Conder, R., Evans, D., Faulkner, P., et al. (1988). An interdisciplinary programme for cognitive rehabilitation. *Brain Injury*, 2, 365–385.

Gordon, W. A., Zafonte, R., Cicerone, K., Cantor, J., Brown, M., Lombard, L. et al. (2006). Traumatic brain injury rehabilitation: State of the science. *American Journal of Physical Medicine & Rehabilitation*, 85, 343–382.

Heinemann, A.W., Hamilton, B., Linacre, J.M., Wright, B.D., & Granger, C. (1995). Functional status and therapeutic intensity during inpatient rehabilitation. *American Journal of Physical Medicine and Rehabilitation*, 74, 315–326.

McMordie, W. R., Rogers, K. F., & Barker, S.L. (1991). Consumer satisfaction with services provided to head injured patients and their families. *Brain Injury*, 5, 43–51.

Niemeier, J. P., & Kreutzer, J. S. (2001). *First Steps Toward Recovery from Brain Injury*. Richmond, VA: National Resource Center for Traumatic Brain Injury.

Osborn, C. L. (2000). *Over My Head: A Doctor's Own Story of Head Injury from the Inside Looking Out*. Kansas City, MO: Andrews McNeel.

Patterson, D. R., & Ford, G. R. (2009). Brain injuries. In R. G. Frank, M. Rosenthal, & B. Caplan (Eds.), *Handbook of Rehabilitation Psychology*. Washington, DC: American Psychological Association Press, pp. 145–162.

Rosenthal, M., Christensen, B.K., & Ross, T.P. (1998). Depression following traumatic brain injury. *Archives of Physical Medicine and Rehabilitation*, 79, 90–103.

Lesson 4

American Psychiatric Association. (2000). *Diagnostic and Statistical Manual* (4th Ed.), pp. 349–356. Arlington, VA: American Psychiatric Association.

Caplan, B., & Moelter, S. (2009). Stroke. In R. G. Frank, M. Rosenthal, & B. Caplan (Eds.), *Handbook of Rehabilitation Psychology*. Washington, DC: American Psychological Association Press, pp. 75–108.

Fann, J., Hart, T., & Schomer, K. G. (2009). Treatment for depression after traumatic brain injury: A systematic review. *Journal of Neurotrauma*, 26, 2383–2402.

Lew, H. L., Poole, J. H., Vanderploeg, R. D., Goodrich, G. L., Dekelboum, S., Guillory, S. B., Sigford, B., & Cifu, D. X. (2007). Program development and defining characteristics of returning military in a VA Polytrauma Network Site. *Journal of Rehabilitation Research Development, 44,* 1027–1034.

Lezak, M. (1988). Brain damage is a family affair. *Journal of Clinical and Experimental Neuropsychology, 10,* 111–123.

Miller, L. (1993). *Psychotherapy of the Brain-Injured Client: Reclaiming the Shattered Self.* New York, NY: W. W. Norton.

Niemeier, J. P., Kennedy, R., McKinley, W. O., & Cifu, D. X. (2004). The Loss Inventory: Preliminary reliability and validity data for a new measure of emotional and cognitive responses to disability. *Disability and Rehabilitation, 26,* 614–623.

Niemeier, J. P., & Burnett, D. M. (2001). No such thing as "uncomplicated bereavement" for clients in rehabilitation. *Disability and Rehabilitation, 23,* 645–653.

Niemeier, J. P., & Kreutzer, J. S. (2001). *First Steps Toward Recovery from Brain Injury.* Richmond, VA: National Resource Center for Traumatic Brain Injury.

Patterson, D. R., & Ford, G. R. (2009). Brain injuries. In R. G. Frank, M. Rosenthal, & B. Caplan (Eds.), *Handbook of Rehabilitation Psychology.* Washington, DC: American Psychological Association Press, pp. 145–162.

Raskin, S. A., & Mateer, C. A. (2000). *Neuropsychological Management of Mild Traumatic Brain Injury.* New York: Oxford University Press.

Rosenthal, M., & Ricker, J. H. (2009). Traumatic brain injury. In R. G. Frank, M. Rosenthal, & B. Caplan (Eds.), *Handbook of Rehabilitation Psychology.* Washington, DC: American Psychological Association Press, pp. 49–74.

Seel, R. T., Kreutzer, J. S., Rosenthal, M., Hammond, F. M., Corrigan, J. D., & Black, K. (2003). Depression after traumatic brain injury: A National Institute on Disability and Rehabilitation Research Model Systems multicenter investigation. *Archives of Physical Medicine and Rehabilitation, 84,* 177–164.

Williams, M. B., & Poijula, S. (2002). *The PTSD Workbook.* Oakland, CA: New Harbinger.

Lesson 5

Brain Injury Association of America. (2007). *The Essential Brain Injury Guide* (4th Ed.). McLean, VA: Author.

Condeluci, A. (1995). *Interdependence: The Route to Community* (2nd Ed.). Winter Park, FL: GR Press.

Ellis, A., & Harper, R.A. (1977). *A New Guide to Rational Living.* North Hollywood, CA: Wilshire Book Company.

Eslinger, P.J., Zappala, G., Clakara, F., & Barrett, A.M. (2007). Cognitive impairments after TBI. In N.D. Zasler, D.J. Katz, & R.D. Zafonte (Eds.), *Brain Injury Medicine: Principles and Practice* (pp. 779–790). New York: Demos Medical Publishing.

Goldstein, K. (1952). The effects of brain damage on the personality. *Psychiatry, 15,* 245–260.

Gottman, J., Notarius, C., Gonso, J., & Markman, H. (1976). *A Couple's Guide to Communication.* Champaign, IL: Research Press.

Karol, R.L. (2003) *Neuropsychosocial Intervention: The Practical Treatment of Severe Behavioral Dyscontrol After Acquired Brain Injury.* New York: CRC Press.

Klonoff, P.S., Lage, G.A., & Chiapello, D.A. (1993). Varieties of the catastrophic reaction to brain injury: A self psychology perspective. *Bulletin of the Menninger Clinic, 57,* 227–241.

Lyons, L. C., & Woods, P. J. (1991). The efficacy of rational-emotive therapy: A quantitative review of the outcome research. *Clinical Psychology Review, 11,* 357–369.

Olkin, R. (1999). *What Psychotherapists Should Know About Disability.* New York: Guilford Press.

Prigatano, G.P., & Schacter, D.L. (1991). *Awareness of Deficit After Brain Injury: Clinical and Theoretical Issues.* New York: Oxford University Press.

Ryerson, S. (2001). Hemiplegia. In D.A. Umphred (Ed.), *Neurological Rehabilitation, 4th Ed.* (pp.741–786). St. Louis, MO: Mosby.

Lesson 6

Bradbury, C. L., Christensen, B. K., Lau, M. A., Ruttan, L. A., Arundine, A. L., & Green, R. E. (2008). The efficacy of cognitive behavior therapy in the treatment of emotional distress after acquired brain injury. *Archives of Physical Medicine and Rehabilitation, 89,* S61–S68.

Caplan, B., & Moelter, S. (2009). Stroke. In R. G. Frank, M. Rosenthal, and B. Caplan (Eds.), *Handbook of Rehabilitation Psychology.* Washington, D. C.: American Psychological Association Press, pp. 75–108.

Ellis, A., & Harper, R.A. (1977). *A New Guide to Rational Living.* North Hollywood, CA: Wilshire Book Company.

Fann, J., Hart, T., & Schomer, K. G. (2009). Treatment for depression after traumatic brain injury: A systematic review. *Journal of Neurotrauma, 26*, 2383–2402.

Khan-Bourne, N., & Brown, R. G. (2003). Cognitive behavior therapy for treatment of depression in individuals with brain injury. *Neuropsychological Rehabilitation, 13*, 89–107.

Lew, H. L., Poole, J. H., Vanderploeg, R. D., Goodrich, G. L., Dekelboum, S., Guillory, S. B., Sigford, B., & Cifu, D. X. (2007). Program development and defining characteristics of returning military in a VA Polytrauma Network Site. *Journal of Rehabilitation Research Development, 44*, 1027–1034.

Lyons, L. C., & Woods, P. J. (1991). The efficacy of rational-emotive therapy: A quantitative review of the outcome research. *Clinical Psychology Review, 11*, 357–369.

Patterson, D. R., & Ford, G. R. (2009). Brain injuries. In R. G. Frank, M. Rosenthal, & B. Caplan (Eds.), *Handbook of Rehabilitation Psychology*. Washington, DC: American Psychological Association Press, pp. 145–162.

Raskin, S. A., & Mateer, C. A. (2000). *Neuropsychological Management of Mild Traumatic Brain Injury*. New York: Oxford University Press.

Rosenthal, M., & Ricker, J. H. (2009). Traumatic brain injury. In R. G. Frank, M. Rosenthal, & B. Caplan (Eds.), *Handbook of Rehabilitation Psychology*. Washington, DC: American Psychological Association Press, pp. 49–74.

Williams, M. B., & Poijula, S. (2000). *The PTSD Workbook*. Oakland, CA: New Harbinger.

Lesson 7

Boss, P. (1999). *Ambiguous Loss: Learning to Live with Unresolved Grief*. Cambridge, MA: Haward University Press.

Doka, K. J. (1999). Disenfranchised grief. *Bereavement Care, 18*, 37–39.

Doka, K. J. (Ed.). (2002). *Disenfranchised Grief: New Directions, Challenges, and Strategies for Practice*. Champaign, IL: Research Press.

Holland, D., & Shigaki, C. (1998). Educating families and caretakers of traumatically brain injured patients in the new health care environment: A three phase model and bibliography. *Brain Injury, 12*, 993–1009.

Kreutzer, J. S., Stejskal, T. M., Ketchum, J. M., Marwitz, J. H., Taylor, L. A., & Menzel, J. C. (2009). A preliminary investigation of the brain injury family intervention: Impact on family members. *Brain Injury, 23,* 535–547.

Lezak, M. (1988). Brain damage is a family affair. *Journal of Clinical and Experimental Neuropsychology, 10,* 111–123.

Man, D.W.K. (2003). Development and application of the Family Empowerment Questionnaire in brain injury. Brain Injury, *17,* 437–450.

Sanders, C. M. (1999) *Grief: The Mourning After* (2nd Ed.). New York: John Wiley & Sons.

Testani-Dufour, L., Chappel-Aiken, L. & Gueldner, S. (1992). Traumatic brain injury: A family experience. *Journal of Neuroscience Nursing, 24,* 317–323.

Woodruff, L. (2008). *In an Instant: A Family's Journey of Love and Healing.* New York: Random House.

Lesson 8

Bauser, N. (2001). *Acceptance Groups for Survivors.* Bloomington, IN: 1st Books Library.

Brain Injury Association of Minnesota. (2009). *Peer Mentor Support Connection Program Policies.* Unpublished document.

Gonzales, P. (2007). *Support Group Facilitator Guide.* Minneapolis, MN: Brain Injury Association of Minnesota.

Lew, H. L., Poole, J. H., Vanderploeg, R. D., Goodrich, G. L., Dekelboum, S., Guillory, S. B., Sigford, B., & Cifu, D. X. (2007). Program development and defining characteristics of returning military in a VA Polytrauma Network Site. *Journal of Rehabilitation Research Development, 44,* 1027–1034.

Lezak, M. (1988). Brain damage is a family affair. *Journal of Clinical and Experimental Neuropsychology, 10,* 111–123.

Rosenthal, M., Griffith, E. R., Kreutzer, J. S., Miller, J. D., & Bond, M. R. (Eds.) (1999). *Rehabilitation of the Adult and Child with Traumatic Brain Injury.* Philadelphia, PA: F. A. Davis.

Lesson 9

Caplan, B., & Moelter, S. (2009). Stroke. In R. G. Frank, M. Rosenthal, & B. Caplan (Eds.), *Handbook of Rehabilitation Psychology.*

Washington, DC: American Psychological Association Press, pp. 75–108.

Cicerone, K. D., Dahlberg, C., Kalmar, K., et al. (2000). Evidence-based cognitive rehabilitation: Recommendations for clinical practice. *Archives of Physical Medicine and Rehabilitation, 81*, 1596–1615.

Cicerone, K. D., Dahlberg, C., Malec, J. F., Langenbahn, D. M., Felicetti, T., K. T., Kneipp, S., et al. (2005). Evidence-based cognitive rehabilitation: Updated review of the literature from 1998 through 2002. *Archives of Physical Medicine and Rehabilitation, 86*, 1681–1687.

Fadyl, J. K., & McPherson, K. M. (2009). Approaches to vocational rehabilitation after traumatic brain injury: A review of the evidence. *Journal of Head Trauma Rehabilitation, 24*, 195–212.

Gordon, W. A., Zafonte, R., Cicerone, K., Cantor, J., Brown, M., Lombard, L., et al. (2006). Traumatic brain injury rehabilitation: State of the science. *American Journal of Physical Medicine & Rehabilitation, 85*, 343–382.

Niemeier, J. P. (2002). Visual imagery training for patients with visual perceptual deficits following right hemisphere cerebrovascular accidents: A case study presenting the Lighthouse Strategy. *Rehabilitation Psychology, 47*, 426–437.

Niemeier, J. P., & Kreutzer, J. S. (2001). *First Steps Toward Recovery from Brain Injury*. Richmond, VA: National Resource Center for Traumatic Brain Injury.

Niemeier, J. P., Kreutzer, J. S., & DeGrace, S. M. (2009). *Choosing, Finding, and Keeping a Job After Brain Injury*. Wake Forest, NC: Lash Associates.

Osborn, C. L. (2000). *Over My Head: A Doctor's Own Story of Head Injury from the Inside Looking Out*. Kansas City, MO: Andrews McNeel.

Patterson, D. R., & Ford, G. R. (2009). Brain injuries. In R. G. Frank, M. Rosenthal, & B. Caplan (Eds.), *Handbook of Rehabilitation Psychology*. Washington, DC: American Psychological Association Press, pp. 145–162.

Ragnarsson, K. T. (2006). Traumatic brain injury research since the 1998 NIH Consensus Conference: Accomplishments and unmet goals. *Journal of Head Trauma Rehabilitation, 21*, 379–387.

Raskin, S. A., & Mateer, C. A. (2000). *Neuropsychological Management of Mild Traumatic Brain Injury*. New York: Oxford University Press.

Rosenthal, M., Griffith, E. R., Kreutzer, J. S., Miller, J. D., & Bond, M. R. (Eds.) (1999). *Rehabilitation of the Adult and Child with Traumatic Brain Injury*. Philadelphia, PA: F. A. Davis.

Rosenthal, M., & Ricker, J. H. (2009). Traumatic brain injury. In R. G. Frank, M. Rosenthal, & B. Caplan (Eds.), *Handbook of Rehabilitation Psychology*. Washington, DC: American Psychological Association Press, pp. 49–74.

Swanson, K. L. (2003). *I'll Carry the Fork! Recovering a Life After Brain Injury*. Scotts Valley, CA: Rising Star Press.

Taylor, J. B. (2006). *Stroke of Insight*. New York: Viking.

Wehman, P., Targett, P., West, M., & Kregel, J. (2005). Productive work and employment for persons with traumatic brain injury: What have we learned after 20 years? *Journal of Head Trauma Rehabilitation, 20*, 115–127.

Willer, B., Rosenthal, M., Kreutzer, J. S., Gordon, W. A., & Rempel, R. (1993). Assessment of community integration following traumatic brain injury. *Journal of Head Trauma Rehabilitation, 8*. 75–87.

About the Authors

Janet P. Niemeier, PhD, ABPP, is an Associate Professor of Physical Medicine and Rehabilitation and Director of Inpatient Neuropsychology and Rehabilitation Psychology at Virginia Commonwealth University Health System (VCUHS) in Richmond, Virginia. She has 25 years of experience in assessment, treatment, advocacy, teaching, and research about persons with brain injury and other disabilities. She has worked to improve quality of life and effectiveness of interventions for this client population in private practice, outpatient treatment facilities, and in inpatient hospital settings.

Dr. Niemeier has a strong record of externally funded research with a primary focus on establishing effectiveness of treatments for persons with brain injury. She currently has support from the National Institutes of Health (NIH), the National Institute of Disability Rehabilitation and Research (NIDRR), and the Virginia Commonwealth Neurotrauma Initiative Board (CNI) to do trials of her methods. Dr. Niemeier has developed comprehensive as well as skill-specific interventions, including the Lighthouse Strategy for improving visual neglect following stroke or traumatic brain injury and a manualized intervention for helping clients get back to work after brain injury. Findings of her trials of these methods are published in first tier scientific journals, giving clinicians the confidence that they are using evidence-based methods in their efforts to enhance cognitive and functional skills for their clients. Dr. Niemeier serves on grant application review committees for NIH as well as the Department of Veterans Affairs, advising committee members about the challenges and needs of persons with brain injury. She is active as a speaker in the Virginia Brain Injury Association and has served as their support group facilitator.

Dr. Niemeier is author of the books, *First Steps Toward Recovery From Brain Injury, Memory Matters,* and *Choosing, Finding and Keeping a Job after Brain Injury.* She has authored dozens of articles in scientific journals, and has been invited speaker for hundreds of national and international conferences, seminars, lectures, papers, and workshops. She is faculty sponsor for the VCUHS physician residents' Journal Club.

Dr. Niemeier is a Fellow, and current President-Elect, of Division 22, Rehabilitation Psychology, of the American Psychological Association. She is also Board Certified by the American Board of Professional Psychology as a Rehabilitation Psychologist and serves as Secretary of the Board. As Secretary she oversees the National Board certification process of Rehabilitation Psychologists.

Robert L. Karol, PhD, ABPP, is president of Karol Neuropsychological Services & Consulting, a group private practice in Minneapolis, MN, specializing in the evaluation and care of persons with acquired brain injury. He was the Director of Psychology/Neuropsychology at Bethesda Hospital in St. Paul, MN for twelve years and was Director of Brain Injury Services.

Dr. Karol co-founded the Brain Injury Association of Minnesota, serving on its Board of Directors for fourteen years and he is a past Chairman of the Board. He has advised the Minnesota Department of Human Services regarding brain injury on its Traumatic Brain Injury Program Advisory Committee, its Neuropsychological Services Ad-Hoc Committee, and its Needs of Adults with Brain Impairment Committee. His work includes having been on the Board of Directors of Accessible Space, Inc., a provider of brain injury residential programming, and on the Advisory Committee of TBI Metro Services, a provider of brain injury vocational services. He served on the Minnesota Department of Corrections Traumatic Brain Injury Expert Advisory Panel. Organizations including hospitals, residential care providers, prison correctional institutions, and insurance companies have utilized his consultation services. He has also taught as an Adjunct Professor at Argosy University.

He is the author of the book *Neuropsychosocial Intervention: The Practical Treatment of Severe Behavioral Dyscontrol After Acquired Brain Injury* and a book chapter about brain injury care: *Principles of behavioral analysis and modification.* His most recent article is *Neurobehavioral Crisis*

Hospitalization: On the Need to Provide Specialized Hospital Brain Injury Crisis Programming. He has given more than 135 workshops, seminars, lectures, and papers.

Dr. Karol is Board Certified by the American Board of Professional Psychology as a Rehabilitation Psychologist and is Certified by the Academy of Certified Brain Injury Specialists (ACBIS) as a Certified Brain Injury Specialist Trainer (CBIST).

Index

Note: Page references followed by '*f*' and '*b*' denote figures and boxes, respectively

Acceptance, 71, 72, 84–88. *See also* Denial; Nonacceptance
  addressing denial, 91–92
  comparison with pre-injury abilities, 93–95
  function of, 84–86
  and identity, 86
  reaching, 95–96
Acute-care professionals, 41–42
Adult children, coping for
  of parent with brain injury, 130–33
    decision making, 132–33
    pre-onset relationships, 133
Al Condeluci, 87
American Psychiatric Association
  Diagnostic and Statistical Manual-IV-TR, 68
Americans with Disabilities Act, 135*n*1
Anger, 71, 72, 76–77
  awareness and, 93
  choosing thoughts, 80–82
  removing, 82–83
  thoughts and, 73–75
Anosognosia, 90
Attention, 30
"Attitude Makeover Questionnaire," 103

Awareness
  and anger, 93
  and grief, 93
"Awful-izing," 109

Balance, 28
Behavioral self-management, 32–33
Behavioral problems, recovery strategies for
  effective communication, 35
  interpersonal relationships, improving, 34–35
  self-assessment, 32–33
"Be Your Own Coach" (BYOC) Strategy, 32–33, 34
Brain injury
  emotional responses to, 55–70, 73
  goals, 8–9
  patients
    people related to, common responses, 113–14
    perception of, 50
  post, symptoms, 25, 58–59
    cognitive problems, 29–32
    emotional, social and behavioral problems, 32–35
    physical problems, 26–29
  rationale, 7–8

Brain Injury Association of America, 117, 155
"Brain Injury Symptom Questionnaire" (BISQ), 25

Cognitive impairments, improving
   attention/concentration, 30
   confusion, 29
   memory, 30–31
   problem solving, 31–32
Cognitive therapies, 48
Communication, 166, 167
   and emotional/social/behavioral problems, 35
Concentration, 30
Confusion, 30
Coping, 99, 114
   for adult children of a parent with brain injury, 130–33
   for employers, 135–37
   for friends, 133–34
   goals, 23–24, 100
   for parents
     of adult children, 122–26
     of married child, 126–28
     of young children, 128–30
   for partners, 120–22
   rationale, 22, 99–100
   for spouses, 114–19
   self-defeating thinking patterns, 101

Daily Information Sheet (DIS), 29
Delayed memory, 30
Denial, 88–96. *See also* Acceptance; Nonacceptance
   and acceptance, 91–92
   organic denial, 90–91
   psychological denial, 89–90
Depression, 68
Diet and restlessness, 28
Disability, 88

Disappointment, 83
Dissatisfaction, 83
Distractibility, 30
Divorce, 119
Dizziness, 28

Ellis, Albert, 75
Embarrassment, 116
Emotional coping, 44–45
Emotional functioning, 33–34
Emotional problems, recovery strategies for
   effective communication, 35
   interpersonal relationships, improving, 34–35
Emotional responses, 55–70
   after losing functions and skills, 67–69
   goals, 56, 72–73
   loss and, 56–57
   rationale, 55, 71–72
   take-home points, 69–70
Employment. *See* Productive activity
Employers, coping for, 135–37
Events, and feelings, 75–76
Executive functioning, 31, 32–33

Family, 32, 34, 116–17
   role of, in rehabilitation, 51–54
   struggling to perceive patient's capabilities, 52–53
Fatigue, 26–28
Feelings
   events and, 75–76
   identification of, 74
   thoughts and, 73–75
Friends, 32, 34, 116–17, 140
   coping for, 133–34

Gait problems, 29
Getting support
   goals, 140

principle, 139–40
rationale, 139–40
support groups. *See* Support groups
"Goal-Setting Scale," 107–8
Grief, 68, 118
awareness and, 93
Guilt, 71, 72, 77–78
choosing thoughts, 80–82
removing, 82–83
thoughts and, 73–75

Healing, 13–15, 59–60

Independence, 86–88
Internet, warning about, 155–56
Interpersonal relationships
and emotional/social/behavioral problems, 34–35
Invisible symptoms, 10–11
"Invulnerability myth," 143

Job search, 165–67

Lower body weakness, 29

Marriage, 119
Medications, and sleepiness, 29
Memory, 30–31
Mentors, 165, 166
Mixed group, advantages of, 147

NAME strategy, 31
Negative outlook, 103
Nonacceptance. *See also* Acceptance; Denial
behavioral symptoms of, 96–97

Occupational therapist (OT), 29
Olkin, Rhoda, 86
Organic denial, 90–91
and acceptance, 92
"Outlook Pitfalls," 104

Pain, 27
Parent Advocacy Coalition for Educational Rights, 129
Parents, coping for
of adult children, 122–26
as breadwinner, 125–26
as nurturer, 123–25
of married child, 126–28
of young children, 128–30
school system, 129
Partners, coping for, 120–22
and family members, 121–22
legal problems, 120
and professionals, 120–21
"Patient Advocate," 121
Peer mentor, 154–55
Peer support group, advantages of, 147
Physical problems, improving
balance, 28
dizziness, 28
fatigue, 26–28
gait problems, 29
lower body weakness, 29
restlessness, 26–28
upper body weakness, 29
Physical therapist (PT), 29
"Pop Psychology," 67
Positive outlook, 103–4
Proactive planning, 163
Problem solving, 31–32
Productive activity
endurance and, 164
interviews, 167
job search and application, 165–67
job stability, 167–68
obstacles and aids to, 165
Professionals, 117
Prospective memory, 30
Psychological denial, 89–90
and acceptance, 92
Psychologist, 44–45

Recovery, 159–68
    brain injury patients, experience of, 162
    goals, 160
    personal plan for day-to-day recovery, 162–63
    rationale, 159–60
    reviewing learned concepts, 161–62
Rehabilitation, 13–15, 59–60
    acceptance of emotional help during, 44–45
    common responses to, 39–40
    getting comfortable in, 45–47
    goal of, 41
    inpatient, 13, 59
    leaving
        coping with, 47
        worried about, 50–51
    nature of, 40–44
    outpatient, 13–14, 59–60
    role of family in, 51–54
    team, trusting, 50
Rehabilitation hospital system, 37–54
    cognitive therapies, 48
    goals, 39
    rationale, 38–39
    real-world responsibilities, 48–49
Rehabilitation therapists, 43
Restlessness, 26–28

Self-awareness, 32
    impairment of, 12
Self-defeating thinking patterns, 101
Self-disclosure, 116
Self-identity
    and acceptance, 86
Self-regulation, 32
Self-talk, negative, 110
Social behavior, 166
Social functioning, 33–34

Social problems, recovery strategies for, 33–34
    effective communication, 35
    interpersonal relationships, improving, 34–35
SOLVE strategy, 31, 34
Spouses, coping for, 114–19
    false comparisons, 114–15, 118–19
    sense of loss, 115, 118
Support groups
    common responses to, 141–42
    drop out, review of, 152–54
    explanation, 142–44
    family needs for, 156–58
    functions of, 144–45
    gains from, 144–45
    issue topics, 145
    online support activities, warning about, 155–56
    peer mentor, 154–55
    selection of, 146
        group facilitator qualities, 148–49
        group structure, 149
        patient preparation, 151–52
        practical considerations, 149–50
        time to start after discharge, 150–51
        types of members, 146–47
    what support groups are not, 145–46

Thoughts, and feelings, 73–75
"3-Minute Chill-Out Technique," 28

Unawareness, 10, 12, 90
Unrealistic expectations, 106
Upper body weakness, 29

Vocational Decision-Making Process Form," 166

Worry, and behavior, 29